contents

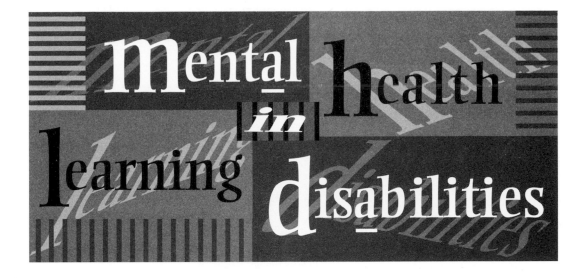

mental health in learning disabilities

A Training Pack for Staff
Working with People who have a Dual Diagnosis
of Mental Health Needs and Learning Disabilities

Edited by
Geraldine Holt and Nick Bouras

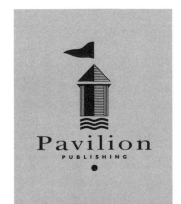

Pavilion
PUBLISHING

Mental Health in Learning Disabilities
Training Handbook

Second Edition

Edited by Geraldine Holt and Nick Bouras

ISBN 1 900600 46 3

Published by:

Pavilion Publishing (Brighton) Ltd.
The Ironworks
Cheapside
Brighton BN1 4GD
East Sussex
United Kingdom
Telephone: 01273 623222

Fax: 01273 625526
Email: info@pavpub.com
Web: www.pavpub.com

This edition first published 1997. Reprinted 1999, 2000, 2001.

A catalogue record for this book is available from The British Library.

Editor: Anna McGrail
Design: Mnich Design Associates
Typesetting and layout: Stanford Douglas
Printing: Ashford Press (Southampton)

INTRODUCTION

Mental health professionals working with people with learning disabilities have seen the move from institutional care to community care, from its inception.

As services have developed, it has become apparent that there is a need for more training on mental health issues to be made available to people working with those with learning disabilities, to improve their skills in recognising mental health needs, managing those problems and, indeed, reducing the risk of their occurrence.

With this in mind, the Second Edition of the *Mental Health in Learning Disabilities* training pack has been fully revised with up-to-date knowledge and information as well as new sections on improving the detection of mental health problems, the mental health needs of children with learning disabilities, autism, and older people.

The contributors all work in the field of mental health, have a variety of professional backgrounds and have been involved with the provision of mental health services for people with learning disabilities.

The chapters of this **Handbook** provide background reading for facilitators of the training modules, and so reflect the professional background from which facilitators are likely to come. Nonetheless, others, including participants in the training modules as well as professionals, who would like to have a basic knowledge of the issues of mental health for people with learning disabilities, will find much to interest and inform them.

The Second Edition of the *Mental Health in Learning Disabilities* training pack is complemented by a video presenting issues highlighted throughout the **Modules** and this **Handbook**.

Geraldine Holt and Nick Bouras.

AN OVERVIEW OF
LEARNING DISABILITIES

Robert Winterhalder

Over the years, successive terms for the condition we currently call 'learning disabilities' have been adopted and then discarded as each in turn became a pejorative label. Of course, there was little wrong with the terms such as mental handicap or mental retardation — the problem lay with the stigma that the condition continued to have in society's eyes. Although some progress has been made in recent years in reducing this stigma, mainly through education and re-integrating people with learning disabilities into mainstream society, prejudices remain. A new term for learning disabilities will do little to improve the situation and will serve only to further confuse both professionals and the public. Indeed, referrals continue to be received by specialist learning disabilities services because someone's son had poor A-level results or a 'patient' has spelling difficulties!

The essential features of the condition now called learning disabilities are a significantly sub-average general intellectual function, accompanied by significant deficits in areas such as social skills, communication, and difficulties in attaining personal independence and social responsibility. The onset of this disorder must be before the age of 18. Traditionally, intellectual functioning has been measured by IQ tests and a significantly sub-average intellectual functioning was defined as an IQ of 70 or below. However, IQ tests are now treated with some flexibility, which permits the exclusion from the diagnosis of learning disabilities of some people with IQs lower than 70 if it is felt that there are no significant deficits in adaptive functioning (the person's effectiveness in areas such as social skills, communication, daily living skills). Learning disabilities can be further broken down into borderline, mild, moderate, severe and profound according to IQ. The IQ level gives an approximate guide to the individual's general level of functioning:

Borderline/mild learning disabilities

This group represents about 80% of people with learning disabilities and their appearance is usually unremarkable and any sensory or motor deficits are slight.

3

In adult life, most of these people are never diagnosed. Most of these people can live independently in ordinary surroundings, although they may need help with housing and employment or when under some unusual stress.

Moderate learning disabilities

People in this group account for about 12% of the learning-disabled population. Most of them can talk or at least learn to communicate and they can care for themselves, albeit with some supervision. As adults, they can usually undertake simple or routine work and find their way about.

Severe learning disabilities

This group accounts for about seven per cent of the learning-disabled population. In preschool years their development is usually greatly slowed. Eventually they may acquire some skills to look after themselves, although under close supervision. They may also be able to communicate in a simple way. As adults, they can undertake simple tasks and engage in limited social activities.

Profound learning disabilities

People in this group account for less than one per cent of the learning-disabled population. Few of them learn to care for themselves, although some eventually acquire some simple speech and social behaviour. As the severity of learning disabilities increases, there is a greater likelihood of sensory and motor disabilities, incontinence, epilepsy, mental illness and challenging behaviour.

It is also important to realise that the variety of terms in use, past and present, reflects the different disciplines and professions involved in this area — each with its own terminology. For instance, mental handicap in the UK (and mental retardation in the USA) are medical terms, whereas 'mental impairment' is a legal term and 'educationally subnormal' is an educational term.

Following a number of scandals in the 1970s, coupled with the enlightened thinking of that period which espoused the principles of 'normalisation', successive governmental White Papers advocated a move away from institutional to community care. Deinstitutionalisation, with the resettlement of people with learning disabilities back into the community and the closing down of the old Victorian learning disabilities hospitals, has been taking place in the UK over the last 10–15 years, although at differing rates in different parts of the country. It is estimated that 70% of the remaining learning disabilities hospitals will close in the next few years. Local services have responded in keeping with the prevailing philosophy governing

4

learning disabilities. This has led to the setting up of different models of care in each locality. For instance, in some areas there are specialist in-patient units for people with learning disabilities who display very disturbed behaviour, whereas in other areas such people are supported in the community with extra resources (although what sometimes happens is that such people may end up being admitted to private units/hospitals out of borough — with all the attendant problems of being far away from family and friends).

There are many ethical and moral reasons why people with learning disabilities should be given the opportunity to live in the community. This basic right — together with others, such as choice — underpin the concept of normalisation. Despite a great deal of thought and planning, it is becoming clear that some errors and misjudgements have been made in certain areas. Indeed, this is not all together surprising when one considers the magnitude and uniqueness of the task in question. This has come about due to inappropriate allocation of resources and funding, often on philosophical/ideological grounds.

Few would argue with the facts that the majority of people with learning disabilities living in the institutions did not need to be there and that their reintegration back into the community has been successful — many of them do not require any form of specialist input whatsoever. However, there is a significant minority of people (possibly up to 40% in all) who have, in addition to learning disabilities, a significant mental health problem. The majority of these people, like their counterparts in the general population, can be assessed and treated in the community. It is also important to realise that institutionalisation can (and does) occur in the community. It is, after all, simply an attitude or a way of thinking and behaving. As such, the principles of institutionalisation can all too easily arise *de novo* within a community placement or be brought in by staff who are themselves moving from hospital-based jobs to community-based ones.

Deinstitutionalisation and reintegration into the community has had far more successes than failures. However, as the fervour of normalisation has begun to settle, one begins to realise the extent to which many people's quality of life has actually deteriorated since resettlement into the community. I can think of several clients who often reminisce about the 'good old days' in the learning disabilities hospital. Certainly, some individuals are far more isolated and vulnerable now than they ever were back in 'the good old days'. One could argue that this is an indictment of the society in which we live and a failure of support services to offer adequate care, but it is also a fact of life. As professionals and carers, we need to be aware of these issues as they can clearly have adverse effects on a client's emotional well-being. Of growing concern in recent years is an awareness that clients with learning disabilities may be even more vulnerable to sexual, physical and emotional abuse in the community (where the abuse may go unnoticed behind closed doors and pulled curtains) compared to the institutions where these acts were more difficult to perpetrate (although of course this did not stop them happening).

Finally, a recent review of research has shown that, despite living in the community, the actual amount of quality time that an individual with learning disabilities spends interacting with the general public and with their environment remains woefully small. There are significant numbers of clients with learning disabilities who are not fully integrated into society. Overall, the material standard of living of people with learning disabilities has increased and they are more satisfied with their services and their life in general. They have increased opportunities to use the skills they already possess and have more choice over daily routine activities. They have more contact with other people and are able to make use of a greater variety of community facilities. They also have more contact and support from care staff and tend to live in a less institutionalised environment although, as we have seen, this is not always the case. However, compared to the general population, these same people remain financially relatively poor and develop few new skills once they have resettled. They continue to show more serious challenging behaviours. There are few, if any, opportunities for choice over life-defining decisions such as where to live and who to live with. They have few relationships with non-disabled people (apart from carers) and receive little active support and quality time from staff.

To finish on a more positive note, great progress has been made over the last 20 years in increasing the quality of life for individuals with learning disabilities. There has been a growing awareness of their psychological and emotional needs and, despite some of the problems alluded to above, the future remains promising.

References and further reading

Emerson, E. & Hatton, C. (1994) *Moving Out: Relocation from hospitals to community.* London: HMSO.

INDIVIDUAL, FAMILY AND SOCIAL ADJUSTMENT

Shaun Gravestock

With the closure of institutions and the development of community support services, most people with learning disabilities will use generic and specialist community-based services to meet their physical health, mental health and social care needs. Thus, any care worker or health professional could be called upon to support a person with learning disabilities in using a variety of community settings and services. This may entail supporting clients, their families, carers, other support workers or professionals, and possibly acting as an advocate for service users.

Contact with unfamiliar people, staff and services may be anxiety-provoking for clients, their usual support network and the unfamiliar people. Yet sensitive under-standing of relevant individual, family and social issues for people with learning disabilities should inform the promotion of client adjustment to community life. A variety of community contacts could then provide positive learning opportunities for all concerned. Changes in societal attitudes and behaviours towards people with disabilities may then follow, in line with the philosophies and processes of normalisation (social role valorisation).

Individual adjustment

Traditionally, people with learning disabilities were considered unsuitable for talking therapies. However, recent psychotherapy work has confirmed the wide range of cognitive, emotional, social and behavioural assets and disabilities found in individuals with 'learning disabilities'.

The key individual issues addressed are described below.

'Intelligence'

Psychotherapy work at the Tavistock Clinic distinguished between cognitive and emotional intelligence, while arguing that there does not seem to be a clear one-to-one relationship between them. Thus, individuals with cognitive impairment on IQ testing may be quite emotionally intelligent, with a deep emotional capacity and preparedness to be in touch with extremely painful emotions.

Also, it may be easier for such individuals to share their feelings given their reduced use of the 'intellectual' defences seen in more cognitively-intelligent individuals. Clearly, the concept of 'intelligence' needs further research to define its several different components and their personal meaning and value to individuals, groups and society as a whole (Stokes & Sinason, 1992; Gravestock & McGauley, 1994).

Personality development

It is unclear to what extent having learning disabilities *per se* may limit an individual's emotional, social and personality development. The bonding and attachment experiences of disabled children with their parents may be inadequate and contribute to difficulties in accepting a disabled child. Early 'maternal deprivation' experiences, parental acceptance and disciplining difficulties have important influences on the later development of internal self-control and self-esteem. Later experiences of failure, rejection, separation, stigmatisation, abuse and dehumanisation may further compromise an individual's personality development (Bicknell, 1983; Waitman & Conboy-Hill, 1992).

However, many people with learning disabilities have positive personality assets, including their capacity to lose, forgive, love, be humble, survive and maintain a sense of humour. Others, such as some people with autistic spectrum disorders, may have severe personality deficits associated with the aetiology of their learning disabilities. Such individuals seem to have little desire to communicate, may not develop a social conscience, have extreme difficulty with relationships and are liable to develop depression in adolescence when their sexuality develops. It should be remembered, however, that all individuals have the capacity for further adjustment and change throughout their lifespan.

Personal insight

Insight into the potentially handicapping situation of being a person with impairments and disabilities is probably more common than society would like to believe. As individuals are expected to function in an ever more complex and competitive society, people with learning disabilities are increasingly made aware of the disadvantages (handicaps) which limit their fulfilment of normal social roles. Such insights may bring a sense of feeling different, frustrated, helpless, sad and angry (Bicknell, 1983; Szives & Griffiths, 1992).

Life events

There are five life events that may be important for people with learning disabilities and their families/carers (Bicknell, 1983):

1   *Diagnosis/labelling* – may be lifelong or inappropriate.

2   *Numerous separation experiences* – may be imposed by respite care and the like, when the individual cannot understand temporary loss.

3   *Breaking of long-term friendship ties* – by resettlement or similar.

4   *Dawning of sexuality* – may herald increased restrictions for individuals with new dilemmas for carers. Parental sexuality and guilt in creating a disabled baby may be linked with the emerging sexuality of a disabled adolescent/young adult.

5   *Bereavement* – individuals may be excluded from the family's bereavement rituals, such as the funeral. Their need to grieve the loss of a friend or relative and often their home, too, may not be acknowledged. This may later lead to depression.

Secondary handicap and defence mechanisms

The defence mechanisms of people with learning disabilities serve ego-protective functions in helping to avoid reality and the experience of sad, painful feelings. Their reactions to 'normality' and our counter-reactions to 'disability' also influence the expression of feelings, attitudes and behaviours within their range of relationships. 'Secondary handicap' is defined as the attacking of intact skills and intelligence as a defensive way of coping with original (primary) handicaps. People may act, walk, talk and behave in exaggerated, overly-handicapped, immature, or over-dependent ways, not only so as to avoid their feelings and issues about primary handicaps, but also to keep the non-handicapped world happy with them (Stokes & Sinason, 1992).

Family adjustment

Over 60% of adults and 80% of children with learning disabilities live with their families. Whilst most families cope extremely well, there is increasing interest in applying understanding of family issues to support the adjustment of people with learning disabilities, their families and carers. Family issues to consider (Vetere, 1993) include the following:

Giving the diagnosis of learning disabilities

The way this sad, bad news is broken to the child's parents is important, as it will affect the family's subsequent sensitivity and adjustment to receipt of other diagnoses and changes in the health and care of their relative with learning disabilities.

Points to consider when giving diagnoses (Ditchfield, 1992) are:

1   *When?*
    Parents/family should be informed as soon as possible, with later reinforcement.

2   *Who?*
    They should be informed by someone they know and trust, and who can cope with their anger and grief.

3   *What?*
    They should be provided with honest information, without excessive confusing jargon.

4   *How?*
    Parents/family should be seen together, preferably with the client, allowing adequate time and privacy, and encouraging questions and the expression of feelings. An honest, empathic, supportive manner should be adopted. The family must be allowed time and privacy to discuss things together afterwards.

5   *Then what?*
    The family should be followed up to reassess their adjustment, to develop their relationships with care workers and professionals, and to promote shared care.

After the initial diagnosis of learning disabilities in their child, the parents should be seen again the next day and at a follow-up home visit within six months. They should be offered early interventions (instruction in home teaching; for example, Portage), practical and emotional support, advice about parents' groups, workshops and so on.

Family bereavement responses

The bereavement response is the psychological work to be done whilst coming to terms with the loss of a significant object or loved person. Such bereavement responses are modified within the families of people with learning disabilities mourning the loss of the perfect child. The continued presence of a relative with learning disabilities acts as a reminder of imperfection and creates extra work, disturbed nights and continued disappointments about failed developmental milestones. After diagnosis, the family members go through some or all of the following stages in their bereavement responses (Bicknell, 1983; Ditchfield, 1992):

1   Initial shock leading to panic, disbelief and denial.

2   Grief, including sobbing, sleeplessness, pain, and projection of grief inwards as guilt or outwards as anger.

3   Bargaining. for example, the family may agree to care for the child assuming the child will walk or talk, with the risk that the child will be rejected should this 'bargain' fail.

4   Acceptance, with the pain subsiding, love re-emerging and reality being grasped.

5   Self-centred and family-centred adjustment work may occur.

6   Other-centred work may occur at a later stage when families may be able to help other families and people with learning disabilities.

Different families and family members work through these stages at different rates and in different ways; for example, mother may achieve acceptance before father, grandparents and siblings.

Additional family life events or crisis points may reactivate bereavement responses and lead to further grief work.

Fixation at various stages may lead to maladaptive bereavement responses, such as anger with professionals, overprotection of clients, chronic family sorrow, disharmony and isolation. Chronic denial may lead to shopping around for second opinions and more acceptable diagnostic labels (such as autism or dyslexia). Prolonged guilt or grief could lead to uncomfortable ambivalence, blaming of the client, infantilisation or overt rejection. Family members and carers may over-identify with disabilities and feel helpless, or engage in frantic activity to cover up chronic feelings of grief, guilt or anger.

Earlier bonding, attachment and acceptance difficulties may lead to an increased risk of abuse by the family or later separation difficulties. Parents may find 'letting-go' even more difficult if earlier bereavement work was not completed, and where there is a shortage of appropriate services. Following the death of a person with learning disabilities, families may require skilled bereavement counselling due to their often mixed feelings (Bicknell, 1983).

Modifications of the family life cycle

Families of people with learning disabilities go through the same life cycle stages as other families. Their additional special transition and potential crisis points requiring family decision-making and reorganisation (Vetere, 1993) include:

1   at diagnosis, when the bereavement response is initiated

2   when hopes have failed; for example, when the child fails to reach developmental milestones

3   when educational, work or placement decisions need to be made by and for family members

4   at puberty or later, when the person with learning disabilities develops his or her sexuality

5   if residential care is needed

6   when parent(s) become elderly or die

7   during future family pregnancies

8   following the physical deterioration or death of the person with learning disabilities.

Family coping and stressors

Family strengths include:

- parental health, energy and morale

- problem-solving skills

- social support networks and material resources

- family beliefs and attitudes towards disabilities.

Family stressors include:

- when the relative with learning disabilities also has behaviour problems, disturbed sleep, poor physical health and multiple disabilities

- financial problems, social disadvantage and isolation

- poor marital relationship

- other relatives with physical or mental illness

- the necessary role adjustments of family members.
  (Vetere, 1993)

It should be remembered that most families want support and advice, preferably from other families and carers, rather than family therapy from professionals.

Social adjustment

The social adjustment of a person with learning disabilities at a given time is determined by multiple changing individual, family, group, service, environmental and societal factors.

The concept of 'handicap' indicates that individuals with impairments and disabilities may experience health and social disadvantages in trying to fulfil normal social roles. In 1976, Nirje, a pioneer of normalisation, described the three 'burdens' carried by people with learning disabilities (Russell, 1985):

1   lack of skills to adapt to the world of work and the social demands of other people

2   lack of resources in society to enable achievement of their potential, but instead social attitudes to disabilities which encourage rejection, segregation and isolation

3   being aware that one is 'handicapped' and the distortions in self-concept and self-esteem that this generates.

Nirje saw normalisation as meaning:

> '*Making available to all mentally handicapped people patterns of life and conditions of everyday living which are as close as possible to the regular circumstances and ways of life of society…i.e. making their life conditions as normal as possible, respecting the degree and complication of their handicaps, the training received and needed, and the social competence and maturity acquired and attainable.*'

Thus, normalisation philosophies regard people with learning disabilities as equal and valued members of society with the right to access valued services. Whilst later simplistic interpretations of normalisation have encouraged treating people with learning disabilities as if they were 'normal', clearly their disabilities and lack of skills differentiate them from average members of society as needing more support, within both mainstream and specialised services. Further, whatever labels are applied to people with learning disabilities, the painful realities of their differences, stigmatised identities and potential social isolation can only be partially ameliorated. Their social coping mechanisms may include trying to pass as normal, denigration and rejection of disabled peers, over-dependence or realistic self-acceptance of their assets and disabilities (Szives & Griffiths, 1992).

Normalisation should be the broad guiding philosophy adopted in planning, delivering and evaluating the quality of services for people with learning disabilities. Service staff and environments should ensure that users accomplish community presence and participation, skills competence, making choices, exercising autonomy and gaining respect (O'Brien, 1986). However, people with learning disabilities should also be supported in achieving realistic self-acceptance (Szives & Griffiths, 1992).

Individualised service packages should ensure that environments are not over-protective or too stimulating. Tailoring the level of staff support to client needs should also allow skills development and risk-taking to increase independence, reduce vulnerability and enhance social adjustment.

Summary

This chapter reviewed individual, family and social factors relevant to the adjustment and self-acceptance of people with learning disabilities, and the promotion of mental health and quality of life in community service settings. This should encourage service staff and professionals to better understand multi-factorial explanations for the development of physical and psychological symptoms, behavioural disorders and psychiatric illness in people with learning disabilities. Sensitive and co-ordinated services will then have the best opportunities to offer appropriate, high-quality support packages to people with learning disabilities, especially those with mental health needs. The future multidisciplinary health care of people with learning disabilities and mental health needs should increasingly include individual, group, family and social therapeutic approaches.

References and further reading

Bicknell, J. (1983) The psychopathology of handicap. *British Journal of Medical Psychology*, **56**, 167–178.

Gravestock, S. & McGauley, G. (1994) Connecting confusions with painful realities: Group analytic psychotherapy for adults with learning disabilities. *Psychoanalytic Psychotherapy*, **8**, 153–167.

O'Brien, J. (1986) A guide to personal futures. In. G. T. Bellamy & B. Wilcox (Eds.) *A Comprehensive Guide to the Activities Catalog: An alternative curriculum for youth and adults with severe disabilities*. Maryland, USA: Brookes Publications.

14

Russell, O. (1985) *Mental Handicap*. Edinburgh: Churchill Livingstone Publications.

Vetere, A. (1993) Using family therapy in services for people with learning disabilities. In: J. Carpenter & A. Treacher (Eds.) *Using Family Therapy in the 90s*. Oxford: Blackwell Publications.

Waitman, A. & Conboy-Hill, S. (1992) *Psychotherapy and Mental Handicap*. London: Sage Publications.

This book includes the following references* as chapters:

* Ditchfield, H. *The birth of a child with a mental handicap: coping with loss.*

* Stokes, J. & Sinason, V. *Secondary mental handicap as a defence.*

* Szives, S. & Griffiths, E. *Coming to terms with learning difficulties: the effects of groupwork and group processes on stigmatised identity.*

EMOTIONAL DISORDERS

Shaun Gravestock and Nick Bouras

The de-institutionalisation movement and community care developments have focused attention on the 20–40% of people with learning disabilities who also have emotional disorders. The broad term 'emotional disorders' is used here to include psychiatric illness, personality disorder, autistic spectrum disorders (autism) and behavioural problems.

This chapter covers the causes, presentations, types and assessment of psychiatric illness, personality disorder, autism, challenging behaviour and selected behavioural disorders in adults with learning disabilities. Understanding 'dual diagnosis' issues should allow learning disabilities and mental health services staff to better address the complex areas of overlap involved in meeting the mental health needs of adults with learning disabilities.

Causes of emotional disorders

Adults with learning disabilities are at increased risk of developing emotional disorders due to the complex interaction of biological, psychological, social and family factors (Russell, 1985). Important factors are listed in **Table 1** overleaf. (See **Chapter II** for further discussion of issues relating to the emotional development of individuals with learning disabilities.)

Professionals and staff unaccustomed to working with adults with learning disabilities may exhibit the phenomenon of 'diagnostic overshadowing'. This occurs when clear signs of an emotional disorder are inappropriately attributed to a person's learning disabilities *per se* and are not seen as giving rise to mental health needs. Alternatively, individuals may be mis-diagnosed as having a psychotic illness when their developmental level has not been fully considered as an explanation for the primitive behaviours, reduced social functioning, and disorganised thoughts and speech which may accompany periods of stress, confusion and change for adults with learning disabilities (Szymanski, 1994).

17

Table 1 Vulnerability Factors for Emotional Disorders

BIOLOGICAL		PSYCHOLOGICAL	
1	Brain damage	7	Personality development
2	Vision/hearing impairments	8	Deprivation/abuse
3	Physical illnesses/disabilities	9	Separations/losses
4	Genetic/familial conditions	10	Other life events
5	Drugs/alcohol abuse	11	Positive/negative learning experiences
6	Medication/physical treatments	12	Self-insight/self-esteem
SOCIAL		**FAMILY**	
13	Attitudes/expectations	19	Diagnostic/bereavement issues
14	Supports/relationships	20	Life-cycle transitions/crises
15	Inappropriate environments/ services	21	'Letting go'
16	Under-/over-stimulation	22	Social/community networks
17	Valued/stigmatised roles/ role models	23	Stress/adaptation to disabilities
18	Financial/legal disadvantage	24	Relationships/resources

Presentations of emotional disorders

The presentation of an emotional disorder in an individual with learning disabilities will depend on his or her usual levels of cognitive, communicative, physical and social functioning, and usual behavioural repertoire, together with past and present inter-personal, cultural and environmental influences.

Generally, the signs and symptoms of emotional disorders presented by adults with mild learning disabilities and reasonable verbal communication skills are similar but less complex than those presented by adults with normal intellect. However, due to their less well-developed cognitive and communication skills, as well as increased risks of physical impairments, adults with moderate and severe learning disabilities are more likely to exhibit disturbed and regressed behaviours and biological functions, physical signs and complaints as presentations of emotional disorders (Fraser & Nolan, 1994).

An individual may present with overlapping signs and symptoms of two or more related emotional disorders at a given time, as the clinical examples below illustrate:

- A man with mild learning disabilities and epilepsy presented with long-standing excessive attention to his personal hygiene due to an obsessional personality disorder, together with recent panic attacks and hyperventilation due to an anxiety disorder.

- A middle-aged woman with Down syndrome and moderate learning disabilities presented with a recent onset of low mood, disturbed sleep and appetite due to a depressive disorder, set against a background of gradually declining social and self-care skills, due to Alzheimer's dementia.

- A teenager with severe learning disabilities, no speech, social indifference, fear of water and finger-flicking since childhood, due to autism, presented with self-injurious and sexually inappropriate challenging behaviours following changes in his daytime activities programme.

Types of emotional disorder

Adults with learning disabilities suffer from the same types of emotional disorder as people with normal intellect. In adults with severe learning disabilities, autism and behavioural disorders are common, but psychoses are often difficult to diagnose when individuals are unable to verbalise complex experiences such as odd ideas and hearing voices. The diagnosis of organic psychoses and personality disorders is difficult in most adults with learning disabilities, as it is hard to obtain an accurate base-line and long-term account of functioning, behaviours and symptoms. The main types of emotional disorders are shown in **Table 2** overleaf.

Psychoses

These disorders are generally over-diagnosed in adults with learning disabilities exhibiting stress-related confusion, odd behaviour, muddled speech and

Table 2 Types of Emotional Disorder

TYPE/ SUB TYPE	PERCENTAGE OF ADULTS WITH LEARNING DISABILITIES	PRESENTATIONS
PSYCHOSES		
Organic dementia	10–25 of those aged over 60 yrs	**Chronic:** confused, forgetful, deteriorating
Alzheimer's dementia	60–70 of those with Down syndrome aged over 60 yrs	
Organic delirium	Not known	**Acute:** confused, agitated, visions
Schizophrenic	} 1–6	Voices, odd ideas/movements, muddled talk
Affective		High/low mood, upset sleep/ eating, regressed
Paranoid		Feeling persecuted, suspicious, hostile
AUTISTIC SPECTRUM DISORDERS (AUTISM)	30	Impairments of social interaction, language and imagination, routines, odd behaviour/movements
NEUROSES		
Depression	} 10–20	Low mood, upset sleep/eating, social withdrawal
Anxiety/phobias		Worries, physical stress, avoidance
Obsessive-compulsive		Repetitive acts/thoughts
PERSONALITY DIFFICULTIES/ DISORDERS	10–20	Chronic maladaptive patterns of behaviour/relating causing distress to self/others
BEHAVIOUR PROBLEMS/ CHALLENGING BEHAVIOUR	20–40	Behaviours that are aggressive, destructive, self-injurious, noisy, socially/sexually inappropriate, resistive, compulsive, stimulatory

suspiciousness. However, individuals with schizophrenic and paranoid psychoses may present with confusion, bizarre behaviours, odd movements, delusional ideas, hallucinations and limited insight.

Affective (manic-depressive) psychoses often run in families and can present as cyclical manic, depressive or mixed disorders. Disturbed activity levels and biological and social functioning often accompany irritability in mania, and bodily complaints in depression. Regression, confusion, vomiting, self-injurious and aggressive behaviours may represent 'depressive equivalents'.

Autistic spectrum disorders

This term denotes a group of pervasive developmental disorders characterised by the triad of impairments of reciprocal social interaction, language and imagination. These social impairments are usually associated with repetitive behaviours and possibly other challenging behaviours and epilepsy. Autism is usually noticed in early childhood and is commoner in males and those with severe learning disabilities.

People with Asperger's syndrome represent a high-functioning variant of autism, with better developed though socially inappropriate language, clumsiness, lack of common sense, and special interests (Wing, 1994).

Neuroses

These disorders are generally under-diagnosed, especially in adults with moderate or severe learning disabilities.

Reactive depression commonly follows the loss of a significant carer, friend or pet, or placement changes, but is often not recognised.

Anxiety states may also develop in response to stress and environmental changes, including resettlement. Anxiety may present with panic attacks, agitation, low mood, pseudo-seizures, and hypochondriacal, self-injurious and acting-out behaviours.

Phobias tend to be over-diagnosed — a refusal to try something new may represent more general avoidance of possible failure. However, specific phobias of dogs, scissors, dirt, water or heights, for example, may occur, particularly in people with autism. The repetitive thoughts and ritualistic behaviours which are resisted and cause anxiety to those with obsessive-compulsive disorder may be mis-diagnosed as autistic features (Fraser & Nolan, 1994).

Personality disorders

Adults with learning disabilities exhibit the full range of personality assets, difficulties and disorders. The diagnosis of personality disorders remains controversial due to their overlap with other emotional disorders and challenging behaviours in adults with learning disabilities. However, chronic maladaptive patterns of behaviour and relating to others, which are not adequately explained by other developmental or emotional disorders, may be best labelled as due to a personality disorder. Whilst personality disorders are more likely to be diagnosed in adults with mild and moderate learning disabilities, similar presentations in adults with severe learning disabilities are more likely to be seen as challenging behaviours. Personality factors are increasingly emphasised in determining suitability for various community placements (Gravestock & Puffett, 1995).

Organic disorders

Delirium, probably under-diagnosed as acute confusion caused by constipation, medication, infections, or epilepsy, is quite common. It may not be noticed and usually resolves with treatment of the underlying causes.

Dementias are increasingly diagnosed as more adults with learning disabilities survive into old age. Roughly eight per cent of adults with Down syndrome aged 35–50 years and 65% of those aged over 60 years will develop Alzheimer's dementia. They may present with loss of skills, social withdrawal, behaviour problems, epilepsy, depression or incontinence. The inevitable functional and physical decline may be rapid. Reduced functioning in ageing adults with Down syndrome may also be due to their increased risk of developing a hearing loss, cataracts, depression and thyroid underactivity (Day & Jancar, 1994).

Challenging behaviours

This term refers to severe and usually chronic combinations of aggressive, destructive, attention-seeking, sexually inappropriate, self-injurious, noisy, hyperactive, and socially inappropriate (for example, pica, faecal smearing or running-away) behavioural disorders. Such behaviours present challenges for service providers as they threaten the physical safety of the client and others, and the client risks exclusion from mainstream services. A significant proportion of adults with learning disabilities and challenging behaviour will have other underlying emotional disorders, including autism (Holt, 1994).

Aggressive and destructive challenging behaviours are usually chronic and often have socio-emotional communicative functions. They may represent attempts to protest, attract attention, express anger, sadness, fear or confusion and even to indicate feeling physically unwell. They are more likely when clients have low frustration tolerance, communication impairments, poor social skills and variable supports. Attention-seeking behaviours may include persistent complaining, crying, bodily concerns and dramatic acts. Sexually inappropriate behaviours include touching and grabbing, stripping, self-exposure and public masturbation. Such behaviours are more often part of a general social disinhibition than due to previous abuse. Other factors in **Table 1** (see p18) may also be relevant.

Self-injurious behaviours occur in 2–13% of people with learning disabilities and are commoner in males, people with severe learning disabilities and people with autism. Such behaviours include skin-picking, biting, scratching, head-banging, face-slapping, hair-pulling, eye-poking and anal-poking, which can cause brain and tissue damage and may become life-threatening. These behaviours may be maintained by complex over-lapping attention-seeking, task-avoidance, socially-aversive and self-stimulatory functions. Physical, emotional and environmental factors can also contribute to the development and maintenance of self-injurious behaviours: for example, earache, constipation, anger, anxiety, depression, under-stimulation, environmental and staff changes.

The term 'challenging' is also increasingly being applied to people with and without learning disabilities who exhibit dangerous behaviours such as fire-setting, assault and sexual offending.

Challenging behaviours may be associated with pica, stereotypies and hyperactivity. Pica is the persistent eating of non-nutritional substances including paper, dirt, hair, paint and cigarette stubs. Stereotypies are repetitive primitive and self-stimulatory movements, such as body-rocking and head-shaking. Stereotypies and pica tend to occur in people with severe learning disabilities, limited mobility, communication and social skills, who are living in impoverished environments. Some children, especially those with severe learning disabilities and language disorders, are hyperactive. They are overactive, impulsive and destructive with a short attention span, but after adolescence, most become apathetic and socially withdrawn.

Behavioural phenotypes

These are repertoires of maladaptive and adaptive behaviours characteristically associated with specific genetic conditions causing learning disabilities. Examples include: Fragile-X syndrome, which is due to repeated abnormal genetic sequences on the X chromosome causing learning disabilities, physical anomalies, speech problems and associated hyperactivity and autistic-like features; Down syndrome, which is due to extra chromosome-21 material causing learning disabilities, physical anomalies and associated obsessive, stubborn and avoiding behaviours; Prader-Willi syndrome, which is due to loss of paternal chromosome-15 material causing learning disabilities, physical anomalies associated with insatiable appetite, gross overeating, obesity, pica, skin-picking, irritability and stubbornness. People with this condition often show angry, aggressive, challenging behaviours if their food-seeking behaviours are thwarted and have personality difficulties, partially due to sensitivity about their physical appearance (O'Brien & Yule, 1995).

Bio-psychosocial assessment

Specialist individualised psychiatric assessment is necessary, given the complex combination of mental health, physical health and social care needs presented by adults with learning disabilities. Psychiatric assessment will consider the client's physical health and social situation, but these areas are more appropriately and thoroughly assessed by their GP or specialist medical doctors and social workers or other learning disabilities service professionals respectively.

The psychiatric assessment process focuses on whether or not the adult with learning disabilities has an emotional disorder; i.e. should the individual be considered as having 'dual diagnosis'? Ideally, the multidisciplinary approach is adopted, whilst also involving the client, carers and other agencies to maximise the gathering of developmental, background, functional, behavioural and observational data. The assessment looks at the client's usual and recent communication skills, functioning, personality, relationships, environments, service inputs, behaviours, medication and physical health (for example, epilepsy) to determine any changes.

The client's verbal communication, hearing and co-operation skills then determine whether their mental-state assessment can include behavioural observations at interview, speech, mood, thoughts, perceptions, orientation, memory and insight about their condition and needs. The client's presenting needs, past and present physical, mental and social functioning are then formulated to try to make a specific diagnosis (if possible) and agree a needs-orientated clinical intervention plan with the client, carers and other agencies (Bouras *et al.*, 1994).

Further professional and carer reports, behavioural observations, blood, urine, EEG, brain scan, chromosomal and psychometric investigations, reassessments in other environments and by psychologists and nurses, and trials of medication and the like, may be arranged as part of the client's ongoing clinical assessment and care plan. Investigations, reassessments and evaluation of interventions over time should determine the client's level of learning disabilities, whether or not the client has 'dual diagnosis', which specific emotional disorder(s) the client has, and whether improvements occur with clinical, psychiatric and other interventions.

Summary

This chapter has discussed the causes, presentations, types and specialist psychiatric assessment of emotional disorders in adults with learning disabilities. As comprehensive local services evolve, psychiatrists have vital roles to play in sharing their skills with diverse staff and professional groups concerned with 'dual diagnosis' issues. Knowledge about the causes can underpin prevention strategies, whilst understanding the presentations and types of emotional disorder will assist those supporting clients to ensure timely access to appropriate services.

Multidisciplinary assessment of adults with learning disabilities and overlapping emotional disorders, including those with autism and challenging behaviours, should resolve historical dichotomisations of behavioural versus psychiatric disorders. In turn, such developments could reduce confusions about clinical and service responsibilities, thus allowing informed assessment of the health and social needs of adults with learning disabilities. Our co-ordinated clinical, supportive and social care inputs will then have the best chance to reduce the adverse effects of emotional disorders on the integration opportunities and quality of life of people with learning disabilities and their carers.

References and further reading

Bouras, N. (1994) *Mental Health in Mental Retardation.* Cambridge: Cambridge University Press.

This book includes the following references* as chapters:

* Bouras, N., Brooks, D. & Drummond, K. *Community psychiatric services for people with mental retardation.*

* Fraser, W. & Nolan, M. *Psychiatric disorders in mental retardation.*

* Holt, G. *Challenging behaviour.*

* Szymanski, L. *Mental retardation and mental health: concepts, aetiology and incidence.*

* Wing, L. *The autistic continuum.*

Day, K. & Jancar, J. (1994) Mental and physical health and ageing in mental handicap: A review. *Journal of Intellectual Disability Research,* **38**, 241–256.

Gravestock, S. & Puffett, A. (1995) Learning disabilities and borderline personality disorder. *Journal of Psychiatric Case Reports,* **1**, 13–18.

O'Brien, G. & Yule, W. (1995) *Behavioural Phenotypes.* London: MacKeith Press.

Russell, O. (1985) *Mental Handicap.* Edinburgh: Churchill Livingstone Publications.

DETECTING AND ASSESSING MENTAL HEALTH PROBLEMS

Steve Moss, Helen Costello and Helen Prosser

Ensuring that people with learning disabilities get appropriate help for their mental health problems is not just a job for psychiatrists. Health and social services staff have an essential role in ensuring that people who have psychiatric problems are identified and referred for comprehensive assessment. This chapter introduces some of the major issues in recognising and assessing mental health problems in this population. In addition, a **Checklist** (see **Handout 2.4**) is included in the **Modules** section of this training pack, designed to help care staff collect information on the mental health of people with learning disabilities for whom they care.

Detecting mental illness in the community

Unlike physical illness, mental illness is partly socially defined, and hence highly interactive with the context in which the person lives. Certain social situations seem more able to contain or deal with the psychiatric symptoms than others, while other social situations may actually produce or exacerbate such symptoms. These factors in a large part determine whether a person seeks professional help for the problem. Once a person has sought treatment, however, the various service providers become the key people in determining whether an individual is referred for specialist help. Each level of service and referral can be regarded as a 'filter' through which some patients will pass and others will not.

For the general population, it is the GP who is the most important filter on the path to psychiatric help. The first visit to the doctor usually occurs when it becomes clear to others that some change has occurred in the person's ability to cope, or in their normal pattern of behaviour. The onset of a mental illness is often heralded by being unable to hold down a job effectively, or being unable to fulfil roles which had previously been carried out successfully; for example, parent, spouse, work. The GP is the one who decides whether the patient (a) has significant mental illness, and (b) whether it can be treated by the GP or whether a referral to a psychiatrist is indicated.

In comparison with this process, many people with learning disabilities have far fewer formal role expectations. They usually do not have spouses or children, and their work roles are often less demanding. As a result, significant depression or anxiety may have no dramatic clearly-defined outward manifestations, although distress to the individual may be considerable. Without specialist knowledge it may be assumed that the symptoms are part of the learning disabilities, with the result that referral to the GP for further psychiatric evaluation may not be made.

The pathway to psychiatric care thus involves at least two steps. Firstly, people who know the individual have to notice a significant change in behaviour. Secondly, the person has to come to the attention of a medical practitioner. Because of the way this pathway works, certain conditions are more likely to be detected than others. Alcohol abuse or schizophrenia are inherently more noticeable than depression or anxiety, because they often result in 'high profile' behaviours which are easily noticed and often cause a nuisance to others. As a result, the people who come to the attention of psychiatric services represent only a fraction of the people with mental illness in the community. For the reasons mentioned above, this difference is even more noticeable in the learning-disabled population. At the time of writing this section, our research indicated that there are probably many people with learning disabilities who have mental illness, but whose problems remain undetected. As a result, they have little prospect of receiving appropriate treatment for their condition. This suggests it is important to focus, not just on the development of psychiatric techniques, but on improving the pathway by which people with learning disabilities gain appropriate treatment. In this respect, the role of care staff in recognising potential symptoms is crucial, since these are the people who are in the best position to identify significant behaviour change, and to make appropriate referrals.

The prevalence of mental illness in people with learning disabilities

In people with learning disabilities, the most common high-profile conditions are challenging behaviours of various kinds — particularly aggression and self-injury. Severe problem behaviours are the most common reason for which people with learning disabilities are referred to a psychiatrist in the UK, accounting for over half the presentations in the long-stay residents, and a third of the admissions from the community. However, these problems are often long-term behaviour patterns, rather than illnesses showing a predictable time course. As such, they often do not fit the established criteria for diagnosable psychiatric conditions. In this respect, the inclusion or exclusion of problem behaviours has a major influence on apparent prevalence. If behavioural disorders are included, the prevalence of psychiatric disorders among people with learning disabilities tends to be inflated.

There is thus considerable uncertainty about the way in which mental illness in people with learning disabilities should be defined for the purposes of estimating prevalence. However, despite the uncertainty, evidence from large-scale studies of morbidity does suggest that, across the spectrum of mental disorder, the pattern of prevalence is somewhat different from the general population. **Table 3** below gives a comparison of two extensive studies of morbidity, one relating to the general

Table 3 Comparison of prevalence figures (excluding dementia) for persons with and without mental handicap

GENERAL POPULATION*		ASSOCIATED DSM IV CODES	MENTALLY RETARDED**	
Diagnostic category	Prev. %		Prev. %	Diagnostic category
Alcohol abuse	5·4	F10·0–10·9	0·0	Substance abuse
Drug abuse	1·7	F11·0–19·9		
Schizophrenia/ Schizophreniform	0·3	F20·0–29	6·3	Schizophrenia/ Psychosis of uncertain type
Autism§	0·04	F84·0–F84·12	3·6	Autism
Manic episode	0·1	F30, F31, F34	1·7	Affective disorder
Major depression	3·2	F32, F33		
Dysthymia	3·7	F34·1		
Phobia	5·1	F40·1, F40·2	2·0	Neuroses
Panic	0·7	F40·0, F41·0		
Obsessive/ compulsive	1·6	F42·0		
Antisocial personality	1·8	Not comparable	10·9	Behaviour disorders

* Bland, Newman & Orn (1988)
** Lund (1985)
§ Ritvo *et al.* (1989)

29

population and the other to the learning-disabled population. It can be seen that the general population shows a much higher prevalence of substance abuse disorders, affective disorders and neuroses. People with learning disabilities are reported as showing higher rates for psychoses and autism, and a very high rate for behavioural disorders.

Problems of diagnosis

How do we know whether a person with learning disabilities has a mental health problem? The answer, unfortunately, is much more complicated than the question. Problems arise when we try to define what we mean by mental illness, and these problems apply as much to the general population as to people with learning disabilities. Before we can learn to detect and diagnose mental illness, it is important to learn something about the basis on which general psychiatry operates.

What is a mental illness? It is perhaps easier to start by comparing it to a physical illness. The diagnosis of a physical condition is often straightforward in the sense that, once all the necessary information is available, the diagnosis can be made with certainty because the criteria are absolute. Thus, conditions like tuberculosis, HIV and syphilis are defined by the presence of an organism. In other cases, particularly at the boundary between physical and mental disease, the criteria are of a somewhat different quality, with the result that treatment and its potential effectiveness are less clearly specified. Thus, conditions like ulcerative colitis are defined by their pathology and others, such as migraine, by their symptoms. Generally speaking, we think of physical illness as something which, in most cases, can be 'fixed'. We go to the doctor, the doctor diagnoses the condition and gives the appropriate treatment.

Mental illness is quite different. Certainly, there are conditions such as dementia which have associated symptoms of mental illness, but these are clearly the result of characteristic brain damage. Similarly, toxic effects due to drugs can produce symptoms of mental disorder, but they usually clear up if the toxicity is removed. Usually, however, we speak of 'mental illness' as something far less clear-cut. The most common mental disorder in the community, for instance, is a mixture of anxiety and depression. It is, of course, highly likely that some people are more susceptible to depression or anxiety than others, but such conditions often relate to life events and general life conditions. For instance, loss of a close relative, divorce, loss of a job. In later life, the sense of increasing vulnerability and reducing status in society can make people particularly sensitive to both depression and anxiety.

Even the very severe mental disorders such as schizophrenia do not have clear-cut biological bases for their origin. True, schizophrenia tends to run in families, so we know there is some genetic component, but genetic predisposition does not seem to be enough to ensure that a specific individual contracts the illness. Also, schizophrenia can have so many different symptoms that a non-expert could easily assume that two cases had completely different disorders. The same goes for depression and anxiety. Some people suffer panic attacks, others lose their self-confidence, others lose their ability to do things they once enjoyed. Frequently, people suffer from a wide range of symptoms relating to a variety of these disorders.

How, therefore, does one decide whether someone has mental illness, and if so, what condition they have? The basic clinical approach is to match the symptoms to various patterns of symptoms which have been found to exist together in mentally-ill people. Thus, in depression, people tend to feel sad or 'down', lose confidence, withdraw socially, feel hopeless, possibly suicidal, and may experience changes in their sleeping and eating. Some or all of these symptoms may coexist in differing levels of severity. In schizophrenia, the classic symptoms include, amongst others, particular sensations of unreality, hearing voices, the feeling of being taken over by an alien force, and delusional beliefs. The exact pattern of symptoms and their particular expression varies from case to case. Also, it is very common for schizophrenia to include symptoms of depression as well. Indeed, depression can, in the most severe cases, sometimes include psychotic symptoms.

Given the complexity of possible symptoms, it is not surprising that even expert psychiatrists do not always agree about the diagnosis of specific cases. Overall, the problem is that there is no simple relationship between symptomatology and diagnosis. Different clinicians show considerable differences in the type and quality of information they try to obtain before making a diagnosis. Some focus mainly on current mental state, some are concerned more with the personality as a whole, while others concentrate on the situation in which the symptoms developed. Many of these differences relate to the clinician's concept of mental illness.

Since the early part of this century it has been clear that an international agreement on diagnosis would be the only way to improve this situation. Two major systems are currently used, the *International Classification of Diseases* (ICD), produced by the World Health Organisation, and the *Diagnostic and Statistical Manual of Mental Disorders* (DSM) published by the American Psychiatric Association. As an example of the way these systems work, **Table 4** overleaf gives the ICD 10 criteria for mild depression.

The use of such criteria make it much easier to gain consensus between clinicians. However, in order to determine whether someone meets these criteria, it is necessary to provide a framework within which information can be systematically collected, and decisions made. People who complete the whole of this training pack will be aware of

Table 4 ICD 10 Criteria for Mild Depressive Episode

At least two of the following three symptoms must be present:

- depressed mood to a degree that is definitely abnormal for the individual, present for most of the day and almost every day, largely uninfluenced by circumstances and sustained for at least two weeks

- loss of interest or pleasure in activities that are normally pleasurable

- decreased energy or increased fatiguability

An additional symptom or symptoms from the following list should be present, to give a total of at least four:

- loss of confidence or self-esteem

- unreasonable feelings of self-reproach or excessive and inappropriate guilt

- recurrent thoughts of death or suicide, or any suicidal behaviour

- complaints or evidence of diminished ability to think or concentrate, such as indecisiveness or vacillation

- change in psychomotor activity, with agitation or retardation (either subjective or objective)

- sleep disturbance of any type

- change in appetite (decrease or increase) with corresponding weight change.

the various areas of functioning which are affected by mental illness. The example of depression has been chosen here because the criteria relate very clearly to a number of these areas. In the case of other disorders, a single criterion may be manifested in a variety of ways, and in this case it is necessary to provide a set of rules to decide whether the observed symptoms are of sufficient clinical significance to meet the criterion. These rules are usually built into the scoring system of the schedule.

Diagnosis in people with learning disabilities

Diagnostic methods for use with this population are not fundamentally different from those used with the general population. However, the poor verbal ability of many people with learning disabilities is clearly an obstacle to psychiatric interviewing. In people who have little on no language, the observation of changes in behaviour can be the first indication of a developing mental disorder. Aggressive acting out, withdrawal, and/or somatic complaints may be observed instead of classic depressive complaints, such as feelings of hopelessness. Clinical features of depression in people with restricted language include somatic symptoms like headache and abdominal ache, hysterical fits, agitation and disturbances of physiological functions such as sleep, appetite and bowel movements. Regressive behaviour is also not uncommon. Detailed information from informants, as well as from the person themselves, is essential. The clinical picture can sometimes be very complicated, especially if a psychiatric disorder is associated with, or concurrent with, an existing challenging behaviour. Evaluating the relative contributions of biological, psychological, social, family and environmental factors to the observed signs and symptoms may thus require repeated assessments over a period of time, and in some cases the use of direct observational techniques. In schizophrenic and paranoid syndromes, where the diagnosis depends on subtle nuances of meaning and experience such as hallucinations and delusional phenomena, the formulation of a valid diagnosis is particularly difficult (Moss, Prosser & Goldberg, 1996).

Rules of good interviewing of respondents with learning disabilities are not fundamentally different from those applicable to the general population. There are, however, two particularly important points to bear in mind. Firstly, people with learning disabilities are more likely to acquiesce to what they believe the interviewer wants to hear. Secondly, they often have a relatively short span of attention. In addition, a wide variety of linguistic and phonological problems can make the respondent's responses difficult to understand. Clinical interviewing of people with learning disabilities is a skill which demands in-depth training and sensitivity to the particular problems faced by these individuals, whether or not they have mental illness.

Recent years have seen the development of a number of instruments designed to improve diagnosis and detection of psychiatric disorders in people with learning disabilities. These include purpose-designed materials such as the *Psychopathology Instrument for Mentally Retarded Adults* (Kazdin, Matson & Senatore, 1983; Senatore, Matson, & Kazdin, 1985) and the *Reiss Screen* (Reiss, 1987). *The Psychiatric Assessment Schedule for Adults with Developmental Disability* (PAS-ADD) (Moss *et al.*, 1993) is a semi-structured clinical interview designed with a multi-level structure to allow interviewing with a wide range of intellectual ability. As such, it provides an

33

assessment system offering different characteristics from brief screening questionnaires, such as the Reiss screen, or instruments relying on informant data and observation only, or self-report questionnaires, or instruments focusing on specific areas of diagnosis such as depression.

Detection of mental illness in the community

As mentioned earlier, a crucial consideration is the need to ensure that people in the community who have mental health problems gain access to the help they need. The remainder of this chapter is concerned with assessment procedures which can be used by care professionals to help them detect mental disorders in the people for whom they care. People living with and working with the individuals are in the best position to notice the kinds of changes which may be symptomatic of mental illness — indeed their information is crucial to a psychiatrist in arriving at a diagnosis. The instrument which is included in this pack reflects this (see **Module Two**). It is a brief screening schedule which is couched in everyday language and very brief to administer. It can be used as a screening instrument or for the regular monitoring of specific individuals who are thought to be at risk of mental health problems when a psychiatric referral is being contemplated.

It is important to point out that this instrument does not cover every aspect of mental health. One important exclusion is that it does not include challenging behaviour. This is a deliberate omission. Challenging behaviours are often long-term behaviour patterns, rather than illnesses showing a predictable time course. Certainly, some people exhibiting challenging behaviour have an underlying mental illness, but equally, there are people with challenging behaviour who probably have no psychiatric disorder. There are many factors which may contribute to challenging behaviour, and it is essential that all these factors are fully assessed by appropriate methods. In relation to the PAS-ADD instrument, the specific focus is on those disorders which are defined as 'Axis I' disorders by the main classification systems, ICD 10 and DSM IV. The instrument may be used with other schedules designed to focus on other areas of functioning (such as challenging behaviour, dementia, substance abuse).

Psychiatric assessment instruments

The Hester Adrian Research Centre at Manchester University has developed a multi-level approach to the assessment of mental health needs in people with learning disabilities. The first two levels of this assessment process — the **PAS-ADD Checklist** and the **Mini PAS-ADD** — can be regarded as 'filters' through which to identify people in the community whose mental health problems may hitherto have been unrecognised. The full PAS-ADD forms the final stage in the referral process and is an in-depth mental state interview, and like the Mini PAS-ADD is designed for use by people who have undergone specialist training. Therefore, only the Checklist will be considered here. The Mini PAS-ADD and PAS-ADD are for use by people who have undergone the appropriate training. Those wishing to explore the possibilities of such training should contact the Hester Adrian Research Centre.

The PAS-ADD Checklist

The PAS-ADD Checklist is the first level of the assessment process. It is an observational screen of behaviours and symptoms commonly associated with mental health problems. The Checklist has two specific uses which will be of interest to those involved in the delivery of services:

(i)   screening populations to identify at-risk individuals

(ii) to enable care staff to monitor changes and patterns in client behaviour by routinely keeping standardised records.

In addition, the Checklist provides a record of mental health which provides background information in any subsequent psychiatric assessment.

The PAS-ADD Checklist is designed primarily for use by front-line care staff or family carers. It is intended to be quick and easy to administer and is written in non-technical language. Carers do not need to have any specific knowledge of mental illness to use it, although we strongly recommend that they have known the person being assessed for a period of at least six months.

The Checklist covers eight broad areas of psychiatric disorder:

● depression
● phobic anxiety
● other anxiety disorders
● hypomania
● obsessive-compulsive disorder
● schizophrenia
● dementia
● pervasive developmental disorders.

It consists of 29 items, each referring to an observable psychiatric symptom. Carers record the presence or absence of symptoms observed during the previous four weeks on a four-point scale:

1   'has not happened'

2   'has happened but has not been a problem'

3   'has been a problem for the person in the past four weeks'

4   'has been a serious problem for the person'.

The Checklist provides three scores relating to different types of mental health problem. Thresholds are provided for each score. People who score over the threshold for any of the three scores should have their potential problem assessed further. The Checklist is designed to be over-inclusive. In other words, it aims to ensure that all potential cases are recognised, but will sometimes identify individuals who subsequently do not prove to have a diagnosable psychiatric illness.

References and further reading

Bland, R. C., Newman, S.C. & Orn, H. (1988). Epidemiology of psychiatric disorders. *Acta Psychiatrica Scandinavica, Vol. 77.*

Kazdin, A. E., Matson, J. L. & Senatore, V. (1983) Assessment of depression in mentally retarded adults. *American Journal of Psychiatry,* **140**, 1040–1043.

Lund, J. (1985). The prevalence of psychiatric morbidity in mentally retarded adults. *Acta Psychiatrica Scandinavica, Vol. 72.*

Moss, S. C., Patel, P., Prosser, H., Goldberg, D. P., Simpson, N., Rowe, S. & Lucchino, R. (1993) Psychiatric morbidity in older people with moderate and severe learning disability (mental retardation). Part I: Development and reliability of the patient interview (the PAS-ADD). *British Journal of Psychiatry,* **163**, 471–480.

Moss, S. C., Prosser, H. & Goldberg, D. P. (1996) Validity of the schizophrenia diagnosis of the Psychiatric Assessment Schedule for Adults with Developmental Disability (PAS-ADD). *British Journal of Psychiatry,* **168**, 359–367.

Reiss, S. (1987) *Reiss Screen for Maladaptive Behavior.* Chicago: International Diagnostic Systems, Inc.

Ritvo, E. R., Freeman, B. J., Pingree, C., Matson-Brothers, A., Jorde, L., Jenson, W. R., McMahon, W. M., Peterson, P. B., Mo, A. & Ritvo, A. (1989). The UCLA-University of Utah epidemiological survey of autism: Prevalence. *American Journal of Psychiatry,* **146**, 194–9.

Senatore, V., Matson, J. L. & Kazdin, A. E. (1985) An inventory to assess psychopathology of mentally retarded adults. *American Journal of Mental Deficiency,* **89**, 459–66.

World Health Organisation (1994) *Schedules for Clinical Assessment in Neuropsychiatry, Version 2.* Geneva: WHO.

THERAPEUTIC INTERVENTIONS

Robert Winterhalder

Over the last 10–20 years, there has been a large increase in the number of different treatments available for various types of mental disorder. The purpose of this chapter is to give the reader an insight into why one type of treatment might be preferred over another in a particular clinical situation. For example, why are some depressed patients treated with ECT, others with antidepressants and others still with cognitive therapy or psychotherapy? Just as physical, psychological and social factors working together contribute to the development of a mental disorder, various physical, psychological and social treatment strategies are available to treat a mental illness. Experience tells us that the best results are obtained when the treatment package encompasses all three treatment modalities, although often it is the case that, depending on the clinical situation, one type of treatment, for example, the use of antidepressant medication or a behavioural therapy intervention, may predominate.

This chapter offers an introductory overview of the indications (and contra-indications) for the various types of treatment available. Further information about these approaches are discussed in the appropriate chapters.

Psychological treatments

These include psychotherapy, cognitive therapy and behavioural therapy (although there are many more in use).

Psychotherapy

In psychotherapy, the therapist tries to help the patient to overcome emotional problems by a combination of listening and talking. In general, listening is more important than talking because the main purpose is to help the patient understand him/herself more clearly. The patient is encouraged to think aloud, which is a good way to clarify ideas that have not been put into words before. It also helps the patient to become aware of links between aspects of feelings and behaviour that have

37

previously been unrecognised. The key elements of psychotherapy include a relationship of trust which allows communication in words, which in turn promotes the understanding and integration of previously unacknowledged aspects of the self and relationships. It also involves finding new ways of indicating and coping with unwanted feelings in order to function and develop more freely and effectively.

An important part of psychotherapy is to restore morale, because most of the patients who are treated have experienced repeated failures and have become demoralised and believe that they cannot help themselves. The release of emotion may be helpful in the early stages of treatment if the patient is emotionally aroused, but it is not generally useful to repeat the process many times.

All forms of psychological treatment include a rationale that makes the patient's disorder more intelligible. The patient may have to piece it together from partial explanations and interpretations (as in psychoanalytically-orientated treatments), or the rationale may be described in detail by the therapist (as in counselling, cognitive therapy and behaviour therapy). Whatever the method of imparting the rationale, it has the effect of making problems more understandable and therefore gives the patient more confidence that he/she can solve their problems. Psychotherapy can occur at many levels, from informal psychotherapy which takes place between friends and confidants to more formal levels of psychotherapy involving professionals.

The unburdening of problems, ventilation of feelings and discussion of current problems with a sympathetic and objective helper occurs at all levels of psycho-therapy. However, they are the core of the less formal psychotherapy and counselling. The aim is to gain relief from the airing of problems and for the client to see them in a clearer perspective when they have talked about them with someone outside the immediate situation. Included in this outer level of psychotherapy is **counselling**, which is another name for a form of psychotherapy offered, usually by non-medical professionals (social workers, teachers and so on), to specific groups of people or for specific problems. For example: marriage guidance counsellors deal with people with marital problems; student counsellors are for students with emotional and academic problems; bereavement counselling helps people who have been recently bereaved. Counselling varies from providing information — for example, about available sources of help in the community — to helping a client understand his attitudes and feelings. The counsellor leaves decisions to the client and withholds direct advice or interpretations. This discourages dependency and so tends to ease the termination of counselling sessions. Counselling is often mistakenly given to people who do not benefit from it, or who would gain as much from support from friends and relatives.

At an intermediate level, where psychotherapy is practised by some social workers and psychiatric nurses, psychiatrists and GPs, problems are clarified within a deepening relationship, unconscious defences are confronted and less conscious motives interpreted when appropriate. Unconscious processes are used to assist psycho-dynamic understanding of the patient.

Finally, at the deepest level of psychotherapy which corresponds to **psychoanalysis**, the therapist concentrates on exploring unconscious motives and anxieties and defences. It encourages the re-experiencing of disturbing early experiences and repetition of this is fostered in order to explore at greater depth the traumas and conflicts underlying the symptoms, which permits regression to the 'child inside of the adult'. Dreams are analysed (they can be regarded as a window looking into the unconscious). This is not encouraged in counselling or the more superficial types of psychotherapy. Repetition or 'working through' is required for clients to resolve conflicts and establish a new way of experiencing themselves and their relationships. The understanding that is sought is more an emotional one than an intellectual one. The aim of treatment at this deeper level is therefore more than symptomatic relief: it is reintegration and change in personality function, both intra-psychic and interpersonal, towards greater wholeness, maturity and fulfilment.

Most of the preceding discussion has been concerned with individual psychotherapy. However psychotherapy can also be carried out within groups, of up to about eight members, in which cognitive and behavioural elements may also exist. **Group psychotherapy** can be used with the intention of bringing about substantial change in symptoms, personal problems or difficulty in interpersonal relationships; as a form of supportive treatment; or to encourage limited adjustment to specific problems. Certain psychological processes take place when people meet repeatedly in a small group to discuss their problems. There is a feeling of belonging to the group, learning from the successes and mistakes of others, discovering that people have similar problems, regaining hope through being valued and helped by others, learning from other members' reactions to one's own social behaviour, copying the behaviour of others and, finally, there is the opportunity to express strong emotions. All these factors are felt to be therapeutic. There is no evidence that the results of group therapy in general differ from those of long-term individual psychotherapy, but it is thought to be well suited to people whose problems are mainly in relationships with other people rather than in specific symptoms. Such groups are often suitable for patients with moderate degrees of social anxiety, presumably because they benefit from the opportunity to rehearse social behaviour. One contraindication, peculiar to group therapy, is that a group should never include a solitary patient whose problem may cause him to be made an outsider (for example, deviant sexual behaviour).

In all types of psychotherapeutic (and cognitive) therapy, the patient **must** be genuinely motivated. The outer levels of psychotherapy, including counselling and supportive psychotherapy, are indicated for those who do not want, or could not tolerate, a deeper exploration and uncovering. People who are reacting to an acute crisis such as bereavement, divorce or loss of a job, whose personality is basically strong and who are capable of adjusting to difficulties, might need only relatively short-term supportive psychotherapy or counselling. At the intermediate and deeper levels of psychotherapy, the main indications are that the individual has a willingness and ability to look at his/her problems in psychological terms. Poor candidates for this level of psychotherapy include people with severe personality disorders and psychosis whose condition may deteriorate further as an attempt is made to explore their unconscious motives and emotions.

In the field of learning disabilities, there has been an ongoing debate as to whether individuals who are cognitively impaired can benefit from psychotherapy. Even in the general population there are many people who are not suitable for psychotherapy: they are not motivated, are unable to see their problems in psychological terms, and so on. It is evident that some people may be intellectually very intelligent, but be unable to see or understand their problems in emotional terms: they find it difficult or impossible to 'get in touch with their emotions'. Conversely, an individual who is less intellectually gifted may have a rich emotional life with which he is fully in touch. Therefore, having a mild to moderate learning disability in itself is not a contra-indication to counselling, or even psychoanalysis, as long as the person understands the purpose of the treatment and is motivated. Unfortunately, some individuals with learning disabilities tend to have 'concrete thinking' (as do some people in the general population); that is, they cannot link their thoughts and behaviour to their emotions, and these individuals are not good candidates for psychotherapy.

Finally, it is generally accepted that people with severe/profound learning disabilities are not suitable for psychotherapy — they may or may not have a rich 'emotional intelligence', but their extremely limited intellectual abilities (often coupled with limited or non-existent verbal skills) mean that a psychotherapeutic approach is not practical. However, other forms of therapy have been developed to address the emotional needs of such individuals. There are non-verbal forms of therapy available, such as art therapy, drama therapy and music therapy. They make use of some of the principles mentioned above, such as trust, ventilation of feelings, and restoration of morale, using different media. In addition, patients who are severely depressed or anxious are unlikely to benefit from psychological treatments in general. This is because their concentration and memory may be poor or they are so preoccupied by morbid thoughts that they cannot make use of the therapist. In these situations, psychotropic medication is generally required first, to improve mood or reduce anxiety to allow the patient to engage with a therapist.

All psychiatric disorders have cognitive (i.e., thoughts) and behavioural components and, for the patient to recover, both elements must change. Behavioural treatment is directed at changing behaviour in psychiatric disorders, but for recovery to take place there must be secondary changes in cognitions. Equally, in successful cognitive treatment a primary change in cognitions must be followed by secondary changes in behaviour.

Cognitive therapy

In cognitive treatment, the therapist attempts to change one or more disordered ways of thinking that characterise the disorder; for example, the irrational fears of a phobic patient or the unreasonably pessimistic ideas of the depressed patient. The aim is to change these ways of thinking directly, with the expectation that other changes will follow. The first step is to identify the irrational ideas: although patients describe some of these ideas, they are usually unaware of others. Next, an attempt is made to change the irrational ideas using several techniques which include teaching the patient to focus away from their distressing thoughts or getting them to question the logical basis of the thoughts they are experiencing. Cognitive therapy can be used in patients suffering from mild to moderate depression, anxiety disorders, panic disorder, obsessional compulsive disorder, and so on. It is clear that, as well as being motivated, the patient must be able to communicate the content of their thoughts to a therapist and have a clear understanding of the treatment process and its aims.

Behavioural therapy

In behavioural therapy, the clinician attempts to alter a prominent behaviour by carrying out an incompatible behaviour: for example, the avoidance behaviour in phobic disorders is treated by encouraging the patient to enter situations he fears (this is called exposure therapy), or unwanted behaviours are ignored whilst more positive socially-valued behaviours are rewarded. Although the ability to communicate one's thoughts and feelings can give valuable information, behaviour therapy can be used in people who have limited or no verbal communication skills. Behaviour therapy will not work if the patient is intent on sabotaging the behavioural intervention plan.

Physical treatments (psychotropic medications and ECT)

When prescribing psychotropic medication, the golden rule is that the benefit should outweigh the side-effects. Of course, this applies to all forms of therapeutic intervention, including psychological and social treatments. If we take depression as our starting point, antidepressants would be considered if the intensity of the depressive episode were moderate to severe. General indications include the presence of 'biological symptoms': loss of appetite with weight loss, insomnia, psychomotor retardation, loss of libido, diurnal variation of mood, and, among women, amenorrhea. They are less usual in mild depressive disorders, but particularly common in the severe forms. Other indications would include the presence of suicidal ideations (although in these cases ECT and the possibility of admission to a psychiatric unit would also be considered), and any psychotic features. Finally, the presence of a strong genetic element which would imply a more biologically-based aetiology to the depressive disorder, a history of previous beneficial outcomes with antidepressant treatment, and the failure of psychosocial interventions in alleviating the depressive disorder would also influence the clinician.

Electro convulsive therapy (ECT) is usually reserved for the more severe types of depressive illness. The two main advantages are that it works relatively quickly (antidepressants begin to lift mood after about two weeks, sometimes longer), and it is a very safe treatment modality with few side-effects. Therefore indications would include situations where a client was acutely suicidal, or had stopped eating and drinking, or was in a depressive stupor — all potentially life threatening scenarios. Other indications would include a persistent depressive disorder that had failed to respond to psychotropic medication, or a previous history of a good response to ECT.

Neuroleptics are indicated in all psychotic disorders regardless of their aetiology. They are able to eliminate or reduce psychotic phenomena in up to 70% of patients suffering from a psychotic illness. They are also used in mania and in challenging behaviour, particularly where a client is over-aroused. Finally, they are also indicated in anxiety disorders as an alternative to antidepressants. In recent years, newer neuroleptics have come on the market, such as sulpiride, clozapine and risperidone. The advantages that these drugs possess over the older neuroleptics, such as chlorpromazine and trifluoperazine, are that they tend to be less sedative and are less likely to cause extra pyramidal side-effects such as Parkinsonism and tardive dyskinesia. In general, these newer drugs are to be preferred unless the patient is over-aroused, when an element of sedation may be beneficial. There is also a reluctance amongst clinicians to use newer types of medication as, understandably, they are less familiar with the effects and side-effects of these drugs and the evidence for the efficacy of the older drugs is more established.

In some cases, it is preferable to administer a drug in the form of a depot preparation which is given intramuscularly once every few weeks. The only types of medication that are currently available in this form are neuroleptics. In other words, there is no antidepressant, anticonvulsant or mood stabiliser which is available as a depot. Indications for using depot formulations instead of oral medication include poor patient compliance or when there is concern regarding the absorption or metabolism of oral drugs. One of the disadvantages of depot medication is that if the patient suffers a concurrent physical illness or side-effects from the depot, the drug naturally stays in the body for several weeks.

Social treatments

A clinician always attempts to elicit which factors predisposed to, caused and/or perpetuated a mental illness in a particular individual. In a social context, factors in the family, at school or at work, in a day centre, and so on, may all be relevant. Once identified, it may be possible to intervene effectively by manipulating the environment. For example, a client may develop an anxiety disorder if their job requirements at work change and the client is stretched beyond their resources. By changing the job requirements to match their skills, the client's anxiety disorder may settle and their confidence and self-esteem grow. Of course if the anxiety disorder persists, further 'environmental manipulation' may be required and/or psychological and pharmacological interventions.

Social treatments can address areas such as housing, financial assistance, education, social activities, family and peer relationships, and so on.

THE USE OF BEHAVIOURAL STRATEGIES FOR PEOPLE WITH LEARNING DISABILITIES

Anna Eliatamby

The 'behavioural approach' is one that many people have heard about, usually in conjunction with Pavlov's dogs. In fact, the approach is very much wider and has a rich technology and a wide variety of therapeutic styles derived from it that can be used to help people with learning disabilities.

The approach can be used to assess a given situation objectively and then propose a suitable intervention, be it for a behaviour problem or for a learning skill. This chapter will describe briefly how such assessments and interventions can be obtained. However, before such a discussion can begin, it is essential to define some of the necessary terminology.

Definitions

Responses are those behaviours that are observable and measurable, i.e. not inferred and which can be described quite clearly in terms of specific and clear criteria. Doing this can help to ensure the effectiveness of any planned intervention and improve carers' ability to be consistent in their reaction to a given response.

A **consequence** is 'an environmental stimulus or event that contingently follows the occurrence of a particular response and as a result of that contingency relationship strengthens or weakens the future occurrence of that response' (Donnellan, La Vigna et al., 1986).

An **antecedent** is similar in form and function to a consequence, apart from the fact that it is an environmental stimulus or event that occurs before a response.

A **reinforcer** is that which is utilised to increase or strengthen the occurrence of a response over time. There are two main types of reinforcer: primary and secondary. Primary reinforcers are those that are naturally occurring, such as food; secondary reinforcers are those that have become reinforcing because of their association with a primary reinforcer.

There are numerous reinforcers that can be used; for example, praise, money and food. Whether or not a particular item is reinforcing is dependent on the perceived value it has for an individual. This can be determined by carrying out an assessment; for example, by asking the person or the carers what they prefer, or by observing the person, or by offering the person a variety of possible reinforcers and recording which one(s) they prefer.

Reinforcers can be used to help people with learning disabilities; for example, to learn to cook a meal. However, it is important to ascertain that the reinforcer is one that is meaningful to the person and is appropriate to that individual: it is of little use to offer sweets to a fifty-year-old man to try to encourage him to learn to wash a car; money would obviously have more intrinsic value. If reinforcers are to be used as part of therapy, then they can be administered in a variety of ways/schedules; for example, immediately, or after a day. (Negative reinforcement occurs when the removal of a certain event results in an increase or strengthening over time of a response.)

Punishment, i.e. presentation of a stimulus which results in a decrease of response rate, has also been used to try to help people with learning disabilities. However, while a variety of techniques — such as electric shock — are available, the questions that need to be addressed are ethical ones: Should such techniques be used to help human beings? Are there not other alternatives that can be used?

These are the basic terms that are used when discussing the behavioural approach. Donnellan & La Vigna (1986) and Evans & Meyer (1989) discuss these terms in much greater detail.

The terms described above are included in quite a range of behavioural strategies; for example, functional analysis, skills teaching, systematic desensitisation and token economies. This chapter will only attempt to introduce the reader to some of these strategies, as they are ones that are most often used to help people with learning disabilities.

Functional analysis

If a person is referred because they have, for example, been reported to be hitting their head against objects, then the first action that should be taken is a functional analysis of the problem. A functional analysis is unlike an assessment that focuses solely on the problem behaviour. It attempts to analyse the function of the behaviour by a thorough investigation of the context in which the behaviour occurs.

There are three main areas to be considered:

- the person who is referred

- the person's situation or environment

- the significant people in the person's life.

Using a variety of techniques, such as questionnaires, interviews and observation, information is gathered. Base-line data on various aspects of the person's life are collected. Carers and/or the person are asked to record the frequency of occurrence of the behaviour and possible reinforcers. Staff may be asked to use ABC (Antecedent, Behaviour and Consequence) charts to try to investigate the behaviour further. With these charts, staff have to record events just before (antecedent) and just after (consequence) the given behaviour occurred. In addition, a diary on the daily activities and information on the person's life history may help in the understanding of the behaviour.

Once the information has been collated and summarised, it should become possible to formulate hypotheses as to the function of the behaviour and hence design a suitable intervention. It is important to remember that rarely does a behaviour have a simple function. More often, a behaviour has a number of functions, and a function may not be related either to the antecedent or to the consequence.

For instance, staff in one particular house noticed that one of the residents began to be upset and aggressive early in the mornings. ABC recordings were carried out but there was no indication of why the behaviour was occurring. Further investigation revealed that one of the resident's favourite presenters on Breakfast Television was on holiday and she wondered why he had suddenly disappeared, as no-one had explained his sudden absence to her.

In general, however, information that is gathered does prove to be useful in formulating hypotheses which can be utilised to construct interventions.

Interventions

Many behavioural interventions can be implemented. The decision as to which one is chosen is dependent on a variety of factors:

- Firstly, the intervention that is designed should be socially acceptable and above criticism on moral or ethical grounds.

● Secondly, people who are going to implement it should participate in its design. This will allow them to state whether they will be able to carry out the plan as well as 'own' it.

In addition, the effectiveness of the intervention should be monitored, for example, by recording the frequency of the behaviour. This enables an objective assessment of whether or not the plan is successful.

Interventions should not be perceived as being able to be applied in the same way to each individual. Each intervention should be adapted to meet the needs of a given situation.

Using a behavioural intervention does not necessarily discount the use of other therapeutic approaches. Other types of therapy, such as counselling, can be used instead of or in tandem with behavioural interventions, as long as those implementing the plan are sufficiently qualified in the given area.

Positive programming

Donnellan and La Vigna (1986) define positive programming strategies as 'a gradual educational process' for behaviour change; a process that is based on a functional analysis of the presenting problems and which involves systematic instruction in more effective ways of behaving.

For example, one man would always start screaming if he was asked to work for a given length of time. He would walk away and then return to the task.

A functional analysis indicated that he was using screaming to indicate that he wanted a break and that he wanted to choose his tasks, such as hoovering, for the day. The alternative strategies that he was taught to use were:

● he planned his day each morning

● he was given a card that he handed to staff to indicate that he wanted a break.

The reinforcer should have positive value for the individual and be one that is age-appropriate and socially acceptable. For example, it is of little use to teach someone to stop hitting people by giving them a Mars Bar every time they do not. Such a scenario may well lead to an obese individual who expects to eat Mars Bars all the time.

Stimulus saturation/overcorrection

Overcorrection is a procedure whereby the individual is encouraged to continue the negative behaviour again and again with the expectation that such repetition will lead to the cessation of the behaviour. It is an aversive procedure and should only be used as a last resort when all other possibilities have been exhausted.

Stimulus saturation, however, is not an aversive procedure. It enables the individual to have access to the reinforcer that is maintaining the desired behaviour.

For example, one man was always searching for a cup of coffee to drink in the factory where he worked. Flasks of coffee were placed at strategic points. This enabled him to realise that he could have coffee as and when he wanted and there was a subsequent decrease in the amount of coffee that he wanted.

Cognitive behavioural approaches

These methods can be used to help individuals who are anxious. They can also be used as part of a systematic desensitisation programme to help individuals overcome fears and phobias. The person, with the help of a therapist, creates a hierarchy of the feared stimulus and is then taught to practise (*in vivo* or in imagination) approaching and coping with each item of the hierarchy while in a relaxed state.

Cognitive behavioural approaches are also used for people with learning disabilities who have problems with anger control. Anger management approaches have been developed and researched by Black and Novaco (1993). These techniques include the client learning to analyse the environmental stimuli that act as triggers for them and to learn self-control techniques that enable them to develop alternative behaviours to each stimulus. Other approaches are discussed in detail by Whitaker (1993).

It is worth using these approaches if it meets the needs of a client, though the technique must be adapted to the needs of each individual.

Some clients may find it difficult to analyse situations that make them angry. I have found it useful to ask clients to draw a cartoon of each stage of the event and then use each picture to discuss the thoughts, feelings and triggers that occurred at that point. This allows the client to discuss abstract issues (thoughts and feelings) in a concrete matter.

Learning new skills

Behavioural approaches have also been used to help people with learning disabilities learn new skills.

The first step in teaching an individual to improve upon a skill is to find out what the individual can already do. A **base-line** of the skill can be formulated by observation.

49

Once the base-line has been ascertained, what needs to be learnt is then identified using a variety of techniques, such as **task analysis**: this enables the task to be broken down into small manageable steps, then an analysis is made of the types of prompts (physical, gestural, verbal) needed to help the person achieve each step.

Once the areas of need have been identified, **teaching programmes** can be written to help the person. A variety of strategies can also be used to help the person practise the task at hand.

One of these is **chaining**, whereby a given sequence of behaviours is taught in a particular order.

For example, to make a cup of tea the first step would be to get all the necessary items ready, such as kettle, tea bag, teapot, sugar, cup and saucer and spoon; the second step might be filling the kettle.

Forward chaining can be used to teach the sequence from the first step through to the last.

Backward chaining, however, is used when there is a particularly complicated sequence of steps to be learned. In such cases, the last step is the one that is learned first: in the above example, this would be pouring the tea into the cup and drinking it.

In some instances it may be necessary to concentrate on one particular step, such as filling the kettle and plugging it in. If this is the case, then the individual with learning disabilities might be expected to practise that particular step a number of times.

Another useful strategy is **shaping**. Sometimes an individual may have a response that approximates the desired one. In these instances, the initial response is rewarded first and this continues until the desired response is obtained. For example, if you want someone to look at you, you would initially reinforce them simply to turn their face toward you. As time went on, it is hoped that the person would begin to look at you.

Summary

Behavioural strategies are based on a rich knowledge-base. They enable professionals to carry out a thorough functional analysis of a problem in an objective manner. This analysis can then be used to formulate hypotheses about the functions of problem behaviours exhibited by individuals with learning disabilities. Once the functions of such behaviours have been identified, a behavioural intervention can be used to help the individual. Behavioural strategies can also be used to help people with learning difficulties learn or improve upon their skills. It is important that all such approaches are only instigated by professionals who have been adequately trained.

References and further reading

Black, L. & Novaco, R. (1993) Anger management: a case study. In: R. A. Wells & V. J. Giannetti (Eds.) *Case Book of the Brief Psycho Therapies*. New York: Plenum Press.

Donnellan, A. M., La Vigna, G. W., Negri-Shoultz, N. & Fassbender, L. L. (1988) *Progress With Punishment: Effective approaches to behavioural problems*. USA: Teachers' College, Columbia University.

Evans, I. & Meyer, L. (1989) *An Educational Approach to Behavioural Problems*. New York: Paul H. Brookes.

Lovett, H. (1985) *Cognitive Counselling for People with Special Needs*. New York: Praeger.

Murphy, G. H. (in press) Understanding aggression in people with intellectual disabilities: lessons from other populations. In: N. Bray (Ed.) *International Review of Research in Mental Retardation*. New York: Academic Press.

Whitaker, S. (1993) The reduction of aggression in people with learning difficulties: a review of psychological methods. *British Journal of Clinical Psychology*, **32**, 1–37.

COMMONLY USED MEDICATION FOR PEOPLE WITH LEARNING DISABILITIES AND PSYCHIATRIC DISORDERS

Yan Kon

Psychiatrists in learning disabilities are clinically responsible for people with learning disabilities who have psychiatric disorders. Some of these people will have serious mental illnesses, such as schizophrenia or depression, and will need medication to treat these illnesses. Others will have emotional problems or behavioural problems which may need the help of medication to calm the situation while the cause of the problem is investigated.

This chapter is concerned with the use of medication: the indications for use, the side-effects to look out for, and how to overcome these. The information given in this chapter is geared to help community workers to understand the basics about medicine so that they can support their clients better, and to help them to recognise when a problem may be medicine-related, and when to contact the general practitioner (GP) or psychiatrist.

Classes

The medicines most commonly prescribed by psychiatrists in learning disabilities fall into the following classes:

- antipsychotics (neuroleptics, major tranquillisers), such as thioridazine

- antidepressants such as amitriptyline

- mood-stabilising medicines (anti-manic), such as lithium

- hypnotic (minor tranquillisers), such as diazepam

- anti-epileptics, such as sodium valproate.

53

Names

Clients and their carers usually know the **proprietary name** of a drug, such as Priadel or Camcolit. This is the name given by the company which manufactures the medicine. These names are designed to be pronounced and remembered more easily. The name used by the doctor is the **generic name**, in this case, lithium carbonate. This is written on the prescription and allows the pharmacist to supply the drug, either Priadel or Camcolit, from whichever company the pharmacy stocks.

In this chapter, the generic names of medicines have been used.

Antipsychotics

Examples:

- haloperidol (Serenace)

- chlorpromazine (Largactil)

- trifluoperazine (Stelazine).

Uses

In general psychiatry, the main use of these medicines is the **treatment of psychoses**, hence their name. Examples of psychotic symptoms are auditory hallucinations, or hearing voices when there is nobody about. People who suffer from these hallucinations may be seen holding a one-sided conversation with empty space. They may also suffer with delusions, i.e. hold a false belief with no basis. For example, they may believe that someone wants to poison them. People who suffer with schizophrenia have psychotic symptoms and antipsychotics are used to treat and manage this illness.

Many antipsychotics have a sedative effect and this is used in the **control of hypomania**. With hypomania, the client is elated, thinks he or she can do anything, is hyperactive and may not sleep for days. The person needs to be treated with antipsychotics until this mood calms down.

In learning disabilities, antipsychotics are often used in the control of **challenging behaviour** like self-injury, hyperactivity or aggression. Antipsychotics sedate the client so that he or she is less likely to react and be disruptive. Management consists of finding the cause of the behaviour and remedying that. Along the same vein, antipsychotics are used in the emergency control of **severe behaviour disturbances** to sedate the client.

These medicines also have a calming effect and are therefore used in the short-term control of **anxiety** while its cause is found and remedied. Unlike some other tranquillisers, antipsychotics are not addictive — that is, people do not develop a craving for them — and so it is not difficult to stop them.

Finally, these drugs are medicines to alleviate certain symptoms which may develop in people who are suffering with **dementia**; for example, anxiety, hyperactivity, delusions, hallucinations.

Side-effects

Unfortunately, antipsychotics do have some unwanted side-effects which must be weighed against their benefits. Sometimes, soon after starting the medicine, clients may develop a **tremor** of their fingers, **dribble** saliva and feel **rigid**, finding it difficult to move. These symptoms are similar to those experienced by people who have Parkinson's disease and are hence called Parkinsonian symptoms. Drugs such as procyclidine (Kemadrin) or orphenadrine (Disipal) are then given to treat these side-effects.

The side-effects may decline with time or if the dose of antipsychotic is reduced. Some antipsychotics are less likely to cause these side-effects. It is therefore important to review medication and to try to stop the procyclidine or ophenadrine, especially as these drugs have their own side-effects, such as dry mouth, gut symptoms, urine retention and blurred vision.

Another side-effect of antipsychotics which may be noticeable soon after starting the medicine is that the client becomes restless and fidgety. This **restlessness** especially affects the legs and has been described as an inability to sit still.

Some of these medicines are worse than others in their ability to lower blood pressure. Patients will complain of feeling **dizzy** when they get up from their bed or chair, and may fall and hurt themselves. The elderly are particularly susceptible. It is important for those who suffer from dizziness to take care. Fortunately, the dizziness usually disappears after the client has been on the medicine for a few weeks.

Abnormal face and body movements may occur soon after starting antipsychotics. Clients may clench their jaw, protrude their tongue, or, rarely, have an **acute dystonic reaction** whereby the client's body is rigidly bent backwards, the head is bent backwards, the eyes are rolled upwards and the tongue protruded. The treatment for acute dystonia is to give an anti-muscarinic drug immediately. If the client has difficulty swallowing, he may need an intramuscular injection of a drug like procyclidine. In that case, take the client to casualty.

Clients who have been on antipsychotics for many years (about 10–20 years) may develop **tardive dyskinesia**, that is, abnormal face and body movements characterised by chewing and sucking movements, grimacing, and slow turning movements of the head and limbs. These are a social handicap that may improve after stopping the medicine. The only treatment is prevention. Antipsychotics should be taken at as low a dose and for as short a time as possible.

It is important to note that antipsychotic medication causes **skin photosensitivity** and pigmentation, which means that the client is more likely to burn in the sun. Thus, clients must apply sunscreen before going out in the sun.

Many people with learning disabilities suffer with epilepsy. Antipsychotic medication tends **to worsen epilepsy** and the anti-epileptic medication may have to be increased to compensate for this.

Clients who are treated with these medicines tend to put on excessive amounts of **weight** because the medicines increase appetite. It may be wise to help clients control their weight.

Choice

Which medicine is prescribed depends on the reason for giving antipsychotics. The medicines differ in their sedative and antipsychotic properties and side-effects.

Depot injections

In addition to the usual route of taking medication orally, some of these medicines may be given by injection into the buttock every two, three or four weeks. They are formulated to be absorbed slowly from this site. This method is good for those who are not reliable with taking oral medication. However, this is not the method to use if the dose needs to be altered frequently.

Antidepressants

Examples:

- older antidepressants: amitriptyline (Tryptizol), dothiepin (Prothiaden)

- newer antidepressants: sertraline (Lustral), fluoxetine (Prozac)

- monoamine oxidase inhibitors (MAOIs): phenelzine (Nardil).

Uses

Some people suffer with a **depressive illness** which may be caused by a lack of certain chemicals in the brain. This is different from just feeling 'fed-up'. Antidepressants treat the chemical imbalance and hence the depression. Only after taking the drug for a couple of weeks will the feeling of depression start to lift. Once the person is well, the tablets should be taken for six months before they are gradually reduced.

Monoamine oxidase inhibitors (MAOIs) are rarely used because they cause dangerous symptoms when taken with certain foods and medicines (see overleaf for more information). People taking MAOIs have to avoid these foods and medicines.

Some people suffer with **anxiety neuroses** whereby they become frightened and panic whenever they see a certain object, such as a spider, or encounter a specific situation, such as tall buildings. They are said to be phobic of that object or situation, and the treatment is to use a behaviour therapy called systematic desensitisation to help them overcome their fear.

Some people are more debilitated by their fear. They are anxious all the time and have frequent panic attacks. They may not even know what makes them panic. In these cases, antidepressants are used to help relieve the anxiety.

Side-effects

Older antidepressants

The older antidepressants tend to be **sedative**. This is beneficial in many cases of depression, where the client is anxious and agitated in addition to being depressed. The antidepressant then calms the client and helps him or her to sleep. In fact, this calming effect becomes evident almost at once, whereas the antidepressant effect takes two weeks to start.

Common complaints include **dry mouth**, **constipation**, **blurred vision** and **sweating**. These medicines also stimulate the appetite which may be an advantage in those who have lost **weight** due to their depression. Like the antipsychotics, they lower the blood pressure and cause **dizziness**, especially when posture is altered.

People who may be already unsteady on their feet, like the elderly and disabled, are particularly susceptible to falls due to this dizziness. These antidepressants may also worsen **heart problems** and cause **palpitations**. In addition, they lower the **epilepsy** threshold and the number of fits may increase.

Newer antidepressants

The efficacy of newer antidepressants is similar to the older ones. The advantage of these newer antidepressants is that they are less likely to affect the heart and blood pressure. Instead of being sedative, they may cause **restlessness**. Some cause **nausea and vomiting** and worsen any **weight loss**. They are also safer in overdose.

With both the older and newer antidepressants, most of the side-effects become less noticeable after a while.

Monoamine oxidase inhibitors

These medicines inhibit the enzyme monoamine oxidase, which breaks down monoamines. Hence, there is an accumulation of monoamines and this treats depression. Unfortunately, some monoamines, when present in the body in high concentrations, will cause a dangerous **rise in blood pressure**. An early warning sign may be a headache. To prevent this possibly fatal consequence, people on MAOIs are not allowed to eat foods, such as cheese or Bovril, or take medicines, such as cough mixtures, with a high monoamine content.

Mood-stabilising medicines

Lithium

There are two forms: lithium carbonate and lithium citrate, and they differ slightly in their activity. They are manufactured by many companies who give them their own company name: Priadel, Camcolit, Phasal, Liskonum, Litarex.

Uses

People who suffer with a fluctuating mood disorder called **manic depressive psychosis** need lithium to stabilise their mood. These people get depressed and need antidepressants to lift their mood, but they may suddenly swing the other way to became manic, needing sedation. To prevent these huge swings in mood, which are so disruptive, clients are prescribed lithium. Although slight fluctuations of mood may still occur, the lithium should cut out the peaks and troughs.

Sometimes a **depressive illness** is resistant to other forms of treatment and lithium may be able to lift this depression. It is also used to lower the mood of those with **hypomania**.

58

In learning disabilities, lithium has occasionally been used to help manage people with **challenging behaviour**, especially if the behaviour problems fluctuate in frequency in line with fluctuating mood.

Monitoring

Lithium is taken on a long-term basis to prevent relapses. It is an effective medicine but has serious side-effects. Before starting on the medicine, clients have base-line tests which include blood tests for kidney and thyroid function. Once the blood level of the drug has been stabilised (0.5–1 mmol/l), blood tests are then done at about six-monthly intervals. If the level is above 1.5 mmol/l, kidney damage may occur.

Side-effects

Side-effects which are immediately noticeable include **nausea, loose bowels, tiredness, hand tremor, feeling thirsty and passing a lot of urine.** These may improve after a while.

Chronic side-effects include **tremor, weight gain, drinking a lot and passing a lot of urine, and slight forgetfulness.** Some people on lithium become **hypothyroid** (that is, their thyroid gland is underactive) and need to be treated with thyroxine.

Toxicity

Toxicity occurs when the blood level of lithium is too high (above 1.5 mmol/l). This may occur if the client becomes dehydrated — due to diarrhoea and vomiting, for example — or he or she is unable to drink a normal amount.

When toxicity occurs, the client may experience the following: **appetite loss, vomiting, diarrhoea, coarse tremor, slurred speech, unsteadiness on his or her feet, sleepiness.** Eventually **coma** and **death** may occur.

Carbamazepine

Uses

Carbamazepine (Tegretol) is used to treat all forms of **epilepsy** except absence seizures. As people with learning disabilities often have more than one sort of epilepsy, carbamazepine is frequently the medicine of choice.

More recently, carbamazepine has been used to stabilise **mood disorders**. Although lithium is thought to be more effective, carbamazepine has the advantage of having fewer side-effects. Sometimes, if lithium is not effective at controlling mood fluctuations, then carbamazepine is added. Connected to this is the use of carbamazepine to control **challenging behaviour**.

Finally, carbamazepine is also used to treat a condition known as **trigeminal neuralgia**, in which the client complains of pain behind the ear and around the jaw joint.

Side-effects

A common side-effect is a generalised **rash**. This is not dangerous and goes away when the medicine is stopped. Some people get **nausea and vomiting**. It is important for carers to look out for signs of **toxicity: dizziness, drowsiness**, and **visual disturbance**, especially double vision. If this is suspected, the client should consult a doctor immediately. If the client develops a **persistent fever, sore throat, rash, bruising** or **bleeding**, consult a doctor immediately. Although rare, this may be a sign of a **blood disorder**.

Monitoring

Taking regular blood samples is now thought to be unnecessary, but it is done to exclude toxicity if it is suspected. In the learning disabilities client group, few are able to articulate toxic side-effects. It may be considered prudent to monitor blood levels to exclude toxicity. Rarely, carbamazepine can cause blood disorders and this, too, can be excluded with a blood test. On the whole, carbamazepine is a safe medicine with few serious side-effects. Hence its popularity.

Hypnotics

Benzodiazepines

Examples:

- diazepam (Valium)

- nitrazepam (Mogadon)

- lorazepam (Ativan)

- temazepam.

Uses

As the name implies, hypnotics are used to **induce sleep**, especially in times of stress. They are useful for a few days, but the cause of the insomnia must be tackled. The danger is that clients can rapidly become addicted to them, experiencing unpleasant withdrawal symptoms when they are stopped.

These medicines have a calming effect and are thus effective at reducing **anxiety**. Note that too much of the medicine will cause drowsiness. The dose has to be titrated so that the client is calm but not asleep. They are useful for a few days while the cause of the anxiety is found and steps taken to remedy the situation, but should not be given for more than a week. They can be used for the control of **acutely disturbed behaviour**, as they are rapidly sedative when given by injection.

Many carers of people with epilepsy will know that medicines like clonazepam (Rivotril) are used to control **epilepsy**. They can also help in the **withdrawal** from other drugs, such as alcohol.

Side-effects

These medicines differ in the length of time they are active. For example, temazepam is active for about eight hours and is therefore useful to help people sleep, whereas diazepam stays in the blood for much longer and is used to reduce anxiety. A common side-effect is **drowsiness** which leads to poor concentration and decreases the client's ability to learn. This side-effect may be dangerous if the client has to operate a machine.

After about a week, the client develops a **tolerance** for the medicine; i.e. the same dose no longer has the desired effect and more has to be taken to get the same effect. The client very quickly becomes **addicted** to the medicine and, although the same dose no longer relieves anxiety, stopping the medicine can make the client feel even more anxious, restless, unable to sleep, sweaty, confused, prone to headaches and craving for the medicine. Weaning an addicted person from hypnotics can be a slow, difficult process.

Taking too much benzodiazepine may cause intoxication; the client may become unsteady, drowsy and may slur their speech.

Anti-epileptics

Different anti-epileptic drugs treat different types of epilepsy. Thus, it is important to know which types of epilepsy your client suffers. A detailed description of the different types of epilepsy is given in **Chapter XI**. Very briefly, there are two groups of seizures, **partial** and **generalised**. The abnormal brain activity that causes **simple partial seizures** arises in a localised or focal area of the brain. The client may complain of butterflies in their stomach, tingling sensation, auras. There is no impairment of consciousness and the client will be able to answer questions. In **complex partial seizures**, there is some impairment of consciousness. There may be abnormal strange behaviours, such as lip-smacking, chewing, fiddling with clothes and the client may seem to be in a trance. This abnormal brain activity may spread to other areas of the brain, resulting in a **secondary generalised seizure**. In **primary generalised seizures**, there is no focal onset. Generalised seizures involve both sides of the body at the same time; for example, tonic-clonic (old term: *grand mal*), myoclonic, atonic, absence (old term: *petit mal*).

The doctor will seldom have the opportunity to witness an epileptic seizure and will have to rely on descriptions given by carers. Accurate information on the frequency, type and time of seizure will help to diagnose what sort of seizure it is, what medication to give, as well as when to give it. Therefore, it is important that carers keep a **record of seizures** and this is brought to the clinic. It may be that seizures tend to occur at a particular time. Medication can be altered to overcome this. Some women experience increased seizures around menstruation and may need extra medication to cover this period.

The **aim of therapy** is to prevent seizures with as little medication as possible. Medication is generally started at a low dose and slowly increased to a dose which controls the epilepsy. However, many of our clients have severe epilepsy which necessitates the use of more than one drug. Similarly, withdrawal of medication should be done gradually, for fear of a rebound increase in seizures. If more than one drug is used, note that nearly all anti-epileptic drugs interact with each other and this alters how the body metabolises the drugs. This is especially important with phenytoin, as it is effective only when the blood level is within a certain range. Another drug may alter its blood level so that it is no longer within therapeutic range.

A few words about **blood tests**: these are done to check the level of drug in the blood. Certain drugs are only effective at certain blood levels — for example, phenytoin — and blood tests can help to decide the dose of drug to be taken. Some drugs have side-effects when the level of drug in the blood is too high — for example, carbamazepine. When epilepsy worsens, it may be wise to check the levels of anti-epileptics. With stable epilepsy, some doctors advise an annual check of blood levels especially as our client group may not be able to tell us about their side-effects. Please note that with some drugs, it is not necessary to check the blood levels because they do not correspond to the effectiveness of the drug. Drugs may have an effect on certain parts of the body, such as the liver, kidneys or blood, and the doctor may decide to order some blood tests to check that these are functioning correctly.

Many anti-epileptic drugs are **sedative**, which can lead to drowsiness and poor concentration. In people with learning disabilities, these drugs can further impair their **ability to learn**. Phenobarbitone is the worst culprit and most people have now been weaned off phenobarbitone and put on newer drugs. In the past few years, a number of new drugs — lamotrogine, vigabatrin, gabapentin and topiramate — have come on the market.

Below are the more commonly used anti-epileptic drugs and their more common side-effects described in alphabetical order. The idea is not to give an exhaustive list but to help carers gain some understanding of the main issues.

Carbamazepine (Tegretol)

This has been covered under Mood-Stabilising Medicines (see p59–60).

Diazepam (Stesolid)

Stesolid is the name of the tubes of diazepam given by rectum in status epilepticus. Diazepam belongs to the group of drugs known as benzodiazepines, which has been covered earlier under Hypnotics (see p60–61).

Ethosuximide (Zarontin)

Uses

Ethosuximide is the drug of choice in absence seizures.

Side-effects

It causes **nausea**, **vomiting** and **drowsiness**, which can be reduced by slowly introducing the drug. It can also cause **behavioural disturbances**. Rarely, ethosuximide affects the **blood**. If persistent fever, sore throat, mouth ulcers, bruising or bleeding develop, contact the doctor immediately.

Monitoring

Drug levels should be checked. Blood tests can be done to exclude blood disorders.

Gabapentin (Neurontin)

Uses

Gabapentin is added to other anti-epileptic drugs to treat **partial seizures**.

Side-effects

Drowsiness, dizziness and **unsteadiness** are common. **Headache, double vision, tremor, nausea** and **vomiting** can also occur.

Monitoring

Unnecessary.

Lamotrogine (Lamictal)

Uses

Lamotrogine was introduced as **add-on therapy** but is now licensed to be used on its own for **partial seizures** and some sorts of **generalised seizures**.

Side-effects

Rash is a common side-effect; the likelihood of occurrence can be reduced with slow introduction of the drug. **Headache, nausea** and **vomiting, double vision** and **unsteadiness** can also occur. Although rare, if the introduction of lamotrogine is associated with a rash, fever, influenza-like symptoms and a worsening of epilepsy, contact the doctor immediately.

Monitoring

Routine check of drug levels is unnecessary.

Phenobarbitone

Uses

Phenobarbitone is used to treat **all forms of epilepsy except absence seizures**. Primidone (Mysoline) is converted to phenobarbitone and this is responsible for its anti-epileptic action.

Side-effects

Phenobarbitone is **highly sedative**. It can cause **confusion** in the elderly. In children, it can cause **paradoxical excitement** and **restlessness**. Drug withdrawal should be undertaken slowly for fear of rebound increase in seizures.

64

Monitoring

Blood tests for the level of drug in the blood can help to indicate the dose a client should be taking.

Phenytoin (Epanutin)

Uses

Phenytoin is a very effective drug used to control **tonic-clonic, simple** and **partial seizures**.

Side-effects

As with most anti-epileptic drugs, clients may feel **sedated**. It is important to watch out for toxic side-effects. The client may feel **dizzy, have double vision, have head-ache** or **be off-balance** when he or she tries to walk. **Frequency of seizures** is also dramatically increased. When toxicity is suspected, contact the doctor immediately. People who have been on phenytoin for many years develop some unattractive side-effects, namely **coarsening of facial features, acne-like rash** and **growth of gums**.

Monitoring

To be effective, the level of drug in the blood must be maintained at a certain level. This can be a problem.

Sodium valproate (Epilim)

Uses

Sodium valproate is effective against **all forms of epilepsy**.

Side-effects

It is generally well-tolerated, although **sedation** can occur. Some people suffer with **gut symptoms**, i.e. nausea, vomiting, heartburn. **Increased appetite and weight gain** is a common problem. Rarely, **hair loss** occurs but this recovers when the drug is stopped. At high doses, **tremor** may occur. Very rarely, sodium valproate **damages the liver**. The client may feel unwell and be jaundiced (skin acquires a yellow tinge); seizure control may be lost. It is advisable to contact a doctor immediately.

Monitoring

Routine blood testing is unnecessary because the level of drug in the blood does not tell us how effective the drug is. However, blood levels are sometimes done to make sure that the drug is being taken.

Topiramate (Topamax)

Uses

This latest anti-epileptic drug is used as **add-on therapy for partial seizures**.

Side-effects

Sedation and **nausea** are common.

Monitoring

Blood level monitoring is not necessary.

Vigabatrin (Sabril)

Uses

Vigabatrin is used in **chronic epilepsy not satisfactorily controlled by other anti-epileptics**. It is used to treat complex partial seizures and tonic-clonic seizures.

Side-effects

Sedation is common. Some people develop **behavioural disturbances** including irritability, nervousness, depression and aggression. Rarely, they may become **psychotic**. Therefore, it may be prudent to avoid using this drug in those with a history of mental illness.

Monitoring

Blood levels are not necessary.

Conclusion

It is important to remember that medicines should be used as part of a management programme. For instance, a person who has a depressive illness may have their mood lifted with an antidepressant but, for the person to make a full recovery, any stresses which precipitated the depression should be resolved. The depressive illness may have caused the person to be anxious and lose confidence; he or she will then need to be rehabilitated back to normal activities.

The medicines discussed in this chapter are a selection of common medicines used by psychiatrists, but by no means all of them. Neither are all the examples of medicines, given in order to illustrate points, the best medicines of their class. Other doctors may prescribe another medicine of that class because they are more familiar with its potency and side-effects, or because that medicine best meets the needs of that particular client.

References and further reading

Kendell, R. E. & Zealley, A. K. (Eds.) (Fifth edition, 1993) *Companion to Psychiatric Studies, Chapter 36.* Edinburgh: Churchill Livingstone Publications.

Levi, M. I. (1993) *Basic Notes in Psychopharmacology*. London: Kluwer Academic Publishers.

Silverstone, T. & Turner, P. (1992) *Drug Treatment in Psychiatry*. London: Routledge and Kegan Paul.

Taylor, M. P. (1996) *Managing Epilepsy in Primary Care*. London: Blackwell Science.

The British Medical Association and Royal Pharmaceutical Society of Great Britain (1996) *British National Formulary*.

CHALLENGING BEHAVIOUR

Theresa Joyce

Recognising and defining challenging behaviour

The term 'challenging behaviour' came into use in the 1980s when major efforts were being made to close long-stay institutions. This was a time when services in the UK were increasingly being planned on the basis of how to implement the values and philosophy encapsulated in the term 'normalisation', as opposed to the previous situation where many of the aims of services seemed apparently more to do with containment and removal from society. Previously, people had been seen as having 'difficult' or 'problem' behaviour — or as being, of themselves, 'difficult' or 'problems'. In that sense, the individuals themselves 'took the blame' for the behaviour. The term 'challenging behaviour' was coined in an effort to redress this balance. Rather than the problem residing in the person, it was instead seen as a challenge for services to overcome.

This challenge was in the nature of the service being able to meet effectively the needs of such individuals. It was recognised that people with learning disabilities would still engage in behaviours which were problematic for themselves or for those around them. Transfer to a community setting, such as a staffed house, would not, of itself, 'cure' problems, although it would hopefully reduce them. It is clear that real progress has been made in the ability of services to understand and respond to clients with challenging behaviour. There is now much greater capacity to deliver services in ways which really address the needs of clients with challenging behaviour — both by reducing the extent of such behaviour and/or ensuring it can be managed if it cannot be 'cured'. Such placements also pay attention to the needs of clients to participate in activities inside and outside of their home and thus focus on more than the challenging behaviour — they also focus on the rest of the client's life. The challenge, therefore, is to respond effectively to clients' behaviour **and** to ensure that individuals have a good quality of life.

So, how do we define challenging behaviour in the circumstances of present-day services? The definition of challenging behaviour is complex. There is no one definition which clearly states and operationalises what is meant by challenging

69

behaviour in a way that makes sense to all those who work with people who challenge. Emerson *et al.* (1987) provide us with a definition which is widely used:

> *'Behaviour of such intensity, frequency or duration that the physical safety of the person or others is placed in serious jeopardy or behaviour which is likely seriously to limit or deny access to and use of ordinary community facilities.'*

However, this definition does not tell us how frequent, intense or long-lasting the behaviour needs to be, nor how much it should restrict access before it can be accurately labelled as challenging. This is because the behaviour inevitably occurs in a social context, and different settings have different levels of capacity to deal with, and tolerance to cope with, behaviour (and the behaviour inevitably occurs in a social context because, if there is no-one else around, there would be no-one to worry about the behaviour or comment on its consequences). Therefore, some settings and some staff will cope with, for example, screaming and self-injury, but will have great difficulty with property damage. Some staff are less worried by inappropriate behaviour in public than others. So, while some behaviours clearly worry people, the extent to which the service is actually challenged in its ability to cope will vary.

Research examining the prevalence of challenging behaviour has encountered all the difficulties in definition outlined above. However, there is a developing consensus on the sorts of behaviour that are likely to be considered challenging. For example, the All-Wales evaluation (Felce & Lowe, 1993) differentiated severely challenging behaviours from moderately challenging behaviours, as follows:

Severely challenging behaviours feature, or include, or are characterised by:

- physical aggression

- destructiveness

- self-injury

- temper tantrums

- wandering off

- antisocial behaviour

- inappropriate sexual behaviour.

Moderately challenging behaviours may feature:

- overactivity

- attention-seeking

- disturbing noises

- objectionable personal habits

- stereotypies.

There is also increasing recognition of the effects of working with such individuals on staff, who can become seriously stressed by supporting people with challenging behaviour, especially in the long term. It is clear that any comprehensive approach to working with challenging behaviour must include not only staff training, but also formally organised staff support (see **Chapter XII**). There is increasing evidence that good management and staff support is crucial if staff are to be enabled to work effectively with clients with challenging behaviour. The ability of a service to provide appropriate support to clients with challenging behaviour will depend on a number of factors. These include many of the features outlined in the *Mansell Report* (DoH, 1993), which suggested that the competence of staff, the commitment of managers, support from specialist staff and good commissioning arrangements are crucial in providing effective services. These attributes would produce staff teams skilled in understanding and responding to challenging behaviour, and managers who provide the necessary support to enable them to do so.

Why does challenging behaviour occur?

The process of deinstitutionalisation has focused attention on challenging behaviour in a way which recognises both the needs of the individual and the complexity of the possible causes of the behaviour. There is now an orientation which assumes that there is a cause for the behaviour and that it is therefore explicable — it is not necessarily random or incomprehensible, or purposely aimed at staff. There has been a move away from medical/biological explanations for challenging behaviour to an explanation which emphasises its social construction. In other words, challenging behaviour is a product of individual factors and the circumstances in which the individual lives, or has lived. It is therefore useful to consider a number of different factors in developing an understanding of challenging behaviour.

Biological causes of challenging behaviour

Some earlier writers on learning disabilities considered that certain behaviours were an inevitable consequence of having that diagnosis. While recognising that not all 'subnormal' people would behave inappropriately, there was also a belief that, when they did, it was not unusual or surprising. Hence medical/psychiatric textbooks could describe 'stable' and 'unstable' defectives and categorise unstable defectives as (for men):

> '...He may pursue his aim by indecent exposure or by violence, crudely
> assaulting elderly women and not infrequently children...'

and (for women):

> '...Women carry on as prostitutes, and become a moral and hygienic menace
> to the street...'

People with profound disabilities could be characterised as:

> 'Some cannot feed themselves and those who do so are so voracious that they are
> in constant danger of choking. Others, like small children, put everything they
> can get hold of into their mouth and swallow it, earth, grass, stones, leather, or
> pieces of cloth and other material torn from their clothes or bedding. Other
> features...are persistent rhythmic movements such as rocking the trunk or
> shaking the head. They may chew their fingers, or indulge in repetitive cries or
> other noises, or have outbursts like temper tantrums. Incontinence and playing
> with urine and faeces are frequent. Most utterances are purely emotional
> expressions comparable to the cries of animals'
>
> (Slater & Roth, 1969).

Many of these behaviours sound very similar to the behaviours described as
'challenging' earlier in this text, such as stereotypy, pica, self-injury.

Increased understanding of both learning disabilities and of behaviour has produced
a less all-inclusive assessment of the likely impact of biological causes on challenging
behaviour.

There are some syndromes which clearly have behavioural manifestations (Lesch-
Nyhan and self-injury; Prader-Willi and overeating), but both of these are rare and
account for a small proportion of the occurrence of these behaviours (Murphy, 1994).

There is also considered to be a link between epilepsy and challenging behaviour
(although clearly not in all cases) and also autism and challenging behaviour.
However, the nature of the link (especially in the case of autism) is not clear and
there are equally powerful explanations which encompass issues to do with learned
behaviour, communication and environmental causes.

Challenging behaviour can, however, have a physical cause. It can be caused by pain
or following illness. For example, persistent pain could lead to self-injury, making
noise, aggression; while the consequence of illness could be refusal to participate in
activities, withdrawal and so on. This could occur due to fatigue as much as any
other cause.

Challenging behaviour as a response to a poor environment

People with challenging behaviour are most at risk of ending up in the poorest quality environments. They are known to be the most likely to be admitted and re-admitted to hospital, and the opportunities for participating in a range of activities are usually restricted for them. Their history, therefore, and (in some cases) present treatment can be characterised by a barren environment with few materials and activities, low levels of social interaction and those interactions being negative and demanding rather than positive and supportive.

Such settings also often ignore all behaviour apart from 'problems', create the possibility of abuse and neglect and restrict access to many things which are important for quality of life (for example, food, activity).

It is clear that the possibilities for developing and increasing behaviours which meet the need for interaction, for food and activity, for stimulation and for the avoidance of unpleasant demands are much greater in these circumstances than in the circumstances of a responsive environment which is geared to providing for a whole range of needs (McGill & Toogood, 1994).

Challenging behaviour as learnt behaviour

Challenging behaviour can be learnt in the same way as any other behaviour can be learnt: by the presentation of rewards following the behaviour. The behaviour may not, initially, occur with the *intention* of gaining a reward, but if an individual engages in a behaviour and there is a consequence which they find pleasant, then they will eventually learn to pair a behaviour with a consequence. (Similarly, if the consequence is punishing, then the assumption is that eventually the behaviour will disappear.)

There are two ways in which behaviour can be rewarded. The first is by positive reinforcement, i.e. something good/rewarding is given; the second is by negative reinforcement, i.e. something unpleasant is taken away.

The things which can be defined as reinforcing will vary according to the individual; for example, cigarette smoking can be a very rewarding activity for one person and totally aversive for another. It is also likely that behaviours will occur in the context of certain setting conditions which can act as a 'trigger' for the behaviour. Hence, staff are often asked to record not only the occurrence of a behaviour, but everything that was going on at the time.

However, understanding what the behaviour achieves for the person and the circumstances which make it more likely to occur is a complex process, and requires careful assessment.

Increasing sophistication in understanding behaviour has enabled staff to move away from simplistic notions which were current in services in the past. At that time, 'problem' behaviour (if not perceived to be random and for no reason) was usually judged to be 'attention-seeking' and often dismissed for that very reason. The underlying assumption that people with learning disabilities should not be seeking attention was usually not acknowledged.

There is now recognition that there may be a range of 'types' of reward which behaviour may elicit. These are broadly categorised as:

- **social**: the reward is interaction with someone else

- **tangible**: the reward is, for example, food or drink — something which can be touched

- **sensory**: the reward is sensory stimulation

- **demand avoidance**: the reward is that the requirement to do something difficult/unpleasant goes away.

  (Emerson *et al.* 1987)

Challenging behaviour as a communicative act

This understanding that there are different types of reward associated with challenging behaviour has led to an acceptance of the hypothesis that such behaviours might have a communicative function. This is especially true in the situation where the individual finds usual methods of communication difficult — if not impossible. As stated earlier, challenging behaviour occurs in a social context and those around the individual will interpret its meaning. This is true whether or not the individual is actually trying to communicate intentionally with another person (the individual may be reacting to an internal state without any intention that this message would be communicated to another).

However, if the challenging behaviour does bring about a response from others that does meet their (maybe unidentified) need, then they might well use it again to get the same response and indeed generalise it to other circumstances in the hope that the same rewarding consequences occur.

For this reason, a great deal of emphasis has been placed on determining the 'communicative function' of the behaviour, and some treatment strategies deal specifically with teaching the individual more appropriate ways of communicating their need (i.e. their desire for a particular reward).

Challenging behaviour as a response to emotional trauma

People with learning disabilities are subject to a range of responses from those around them, some of which may be supportive and some of which may be abusive. The abuse can be physical, sexual or emotional, and all of these will have an effect on the individual. It is now also recognised that people can and do find their disabilities painful to cope with (Sinason, 1992). Some challenging behaviours can be traced back to situations where the individual has been abused, and it is useful to remember that verbal abuse (for example, name-calling and being laughed at) is not an uncommon experience for people with learning disabilities. It is also important to remember that people with learning disabilities are vulnerable to sexual abuse (Turk & Brown, 1993). Challenging behaviour can be a response to this trauma.

Challenging behaviour can also be an expression of anger or misery or pain at the fact of being disabled and the life experiences to which it has led.

Challenging behaviour in relation to a mental illness

People with learning disabilities can also suffer from a mental illness which can affect their behaviour. It is important to exclude diagnosable mental illness as a cause of challenging behaviour.

How to assess the causes and functions of challenging behaviour

The previous section outlined possible causes of challenging behaviour. This section will consider how to assess those causes, and it is clear that there is unlikely to be one simple 'cause'.

In order to assess behaviour, the behaviour(s) that we are interested in must be clearly defined: for instance, 'aggression' and 'self-injury' do not give a picture of what actually does occur. Different behaviours may have the same function and the same behaviour can have different functions. For example, one client used self-injury frequently in order to obtain a cup of tea; however, she also occasionally used self-injury to be removed from an environment which she found to be too noisy. A full analysis will nevertheless require much more than noting when the behaviour occurs.

75

Many individuals have more than one challenging behaviour, therefore each behaviour needs to be considered separately.

The main methods of assessing challenging behaviour have a number of components. They require examination of the individual's **history**, especially in terms of previous interventions and placements (this helps determine if previous environments may have played a part in the development of the behaviour). Assessment of the **environment** — for example, in terms of routines, activities, staff and other clients — is important, and also assessment of the **target behaviours**, both in terms of antecedents and consequences. It is also important to assess **reinforcers** or rewards for the individual (for example, with the help of an instrument such as the *Reinforcement Inventory for Adults,* Willis & LaVigna, 1985).

This type of comprehensive assessment is often called **functional analysis**, as it implies that not only is the behaviour assessed, but also as many as possible of the variables or factors which might contribute to it. In other words, we are seeking to discover what *purpose* a behaviour serves for that specific person. It is essentially an individualistic approach and requires careful observation and good knowledge of the individual and his or her life.

Functional analysis is, therefore, much more complex than the sorts of assessment which were routinely undertaken previously. Staff will be asked to keep **records**, but they are unlikely to be the main or sole source of information about the circumstances in which the challenging behaviour occurs. Analysis of challenging behaviour should no longer be based simply on ABC charts (antecedent, behaviour and consequence), although such information will still be necessary.

There are now a number of **structured instruments** available to gather relevant information. An example of such an instrument is the *Behaviour Assessment Guide* (Willis, La Vigna & Donnellan, 1987).

Assessment will also require **observation**. This is increasingly being carried out with the aid of microcomputers which have been programmed so that observed behaviour can be categorised according to the type of behaviour which is occurring, and to do this at pre-determined intervals (often between 10 and 30 seconds). The behaviours have been categorised to reflect behaviours relevant to the analysis. For example, it is possible to note when clients are doing nothing, at what point they receive activity or interaction, and at what point in this stream of behaviour the challenging behaviour occurs. It is therefore possible to determine whether the challenging behaviour follows, for example, a long period of inactivity and whether it is responded to by interaction or by an activity or perhaps food; or whether the challenging behaviour follows an activity or request to carry out a task. These observations are carried out in the natural setting.

It may not always be possible to gather sufficient data in the natural setting, and in these circumstances special settings are produced which might mirror the sorts of situations where the challenging behaviour occurs. These are known as analogue conditions and are described by Iwata *et al.* (1982) in an analysis of self-injurious behaviour.

After assessment

Then what? Ways of responding to challenging behaviour

Assessment focuses on both the individual and the environment to determine the function of the behaviour — and responses to the behaviour also need to focus on these issues. There is now a body of knowledge about how we can organise **environments** so that at least some of the features implicated in the production of challenging behaviour can be addressed. McGill and Toogood (1994) provide a summary of the way in which characteristics of the environment can maintain challenging behaviour and point out which features should be present in a high-quality setting which will work to reduce challenging behaviour.

Behaviour maintained by:	Environment characterised by:
Escape or avoidance of aversive situations	Intermittently high levels of overt and covert social control and abuse
Increased social contact	Low levels of social contact
Adjustment of levels of sensory stimulation	Barren, unstimulating environment
Increased access to preferred objects and activities (tangible reinforcement).	Regimes which rigidly control access to preferred objects/activities.

(From: Providing Helpful Environments. In: Emerson, McGill & Mansell (Eds.) (1994) *Challenging Behaviour: Designing high quality services.*)

This summary of the way in which environments can actually mediate the production of challenging behaviour provides clear direction for the way in which environments can be helpful.

77

Environments need to provide:

- good levels of positive interaction, which can be based around appropriate rather than inappropriate behaviour

- support in activities

- a range of activities and materials which are relevant and meaningful.

This clearly all needs organisation and management. It is not helpful if activities occur on an *ad hoc* or unpredictable basis, and if the support to participate in them is inconsistent.

Attention can also be paid to possible triggers in the environment and action taken to reduce them, for example, high levels of noise. How many times have there been situations where people are talking, the television is on and the radio in another room, and the washing machine? The aim is to produce an environment in which constructive activity is planned and available, and in which inappropriate behaviour can be replaced, over time, with more appropriate alternatives.

In addition to attending to the environment, it is also important to focus on specific ways of working with the individual. This may encompass two aspects — **reactive strategies** and **treatment**.

Prior to the growth of behaviour analysis, the 'treatment' for challenging behaviour was behaviour modification. Many of the responses to the behaviour were 'punishing' — the assumption being that if the consequences for the client were 'unpleasant', then the behaviour would be suppressed. However, in the absence of sophisticated understanding of what each individual found rewarding or punishing, and in the absence of understanding the function of the behaviour, then many staff working with people with challenging behaviour adopted simplistic solutions to all behaviour.

Therefore, behaviour was often described as 'attention-seeking', and the response was to ignore it. This was based on the assumption that, if the behaviour was not rewarded, it would disappear. Sometimes, more active strategies were used; for example, aggression was often responded to by time-out or by seclusion. This would have a punishing effect if the function of the behaviour was to get attention. However, if the function of the behaviour was to *avoid* an activity or a situation, then time-out (by removing the demand) would actually reinforce the behaviour.

Non-aversive interventions

Recent years have also seen increasing emphasis on using 'non-aversive' strategies as a means of working with people with challenging behaviour. This developed from a 'values' perspective which emphasises the importance of valued social roles for people with disabilities and which recognises their right to be treated with respect. The history of institutional care is one where punishment/aversive strategies were the most common means of responding to challenging behaviour. This raises ethical issues, especially where the client is dependent on staff and where staff have a lot of power in determining what happens to the client. A wide range of aversive strategies have been used in the past — including seclusion, noxious tastes, electric shock. The aim now is to use non-aversive or non-punishing methods of responding to behaviour by creating positive opportunities for participation in activity and for learning, and by rewarding appropriate behaviour instead of focusing on punishing inappropriate behaviour.

Reinforcement can be delivered in a manner which develops more appropriate behaviours — either by reinforcing non-occurrence of the challenging behaviour and/or by reinforcing other behaviours which are more appropriate. For example, if an individual challenges services by perhaps screaming, then staff could deliver reinforcement for specific periods of time when screaming does not occur; they could deliver reinforcement when appropriate language or communication occurred; and they could try to teach more appropriate methods of communicating the need presently being expressed by screaming.

In addition to using reinforcement as a means of helping people develop more appropriate behaviours, individuals with challenging behaviour may also find that being taught to relax in stressful situations or when they get anxious is useful. A psychotherapeutic approach can also be useful in terms of being able to help individuals cope with the pain of their disability.

As well as providing a helpful environment, teaching new skills and structuring reinforcement to help replace behaviours, staff also need to know how to respond when the behaviour does occur. Challenging behaviour does not disappear overnight and, in many cases, does not disappear completely at all. There needs to be a clearly worked out reactive strategy (King, 1995), which may go through a series of stages. These may include a range of interruption strategies such as redirection, instructional control, assisting the person to relax, and so on. Giving PRN medication may also be part of a reactive strategy and, hopefully not frequently, breakaway and/or control and restraint procedures. If restraint procedures are to be used, then all staff need to be trained in them by an instructor qualified to do so, and they need to be regularly reviewed and monitored.

It needs to be clearly understood that these are not treatment strategies, they are instead a way of coping with the situation through a series of stages.

For example, a strategy for one client was firstly to try to redirect her from her challenging behaviour into another activity. (This client would typically try to hit staff.) If unsuccessful, the staff instructed her to (for example): 'Put your hands by your sides'. The instructions were **positively phrased**: they told the client what to do, instead of what not to do. (In this case, staff stopped saying: 'Don't hit me'.)

Medication when required (PRN) was given at a clearly defined stage. In this way it became less necessary for staff to have to resort to breakaway techniques as they became more skilled in defusing potentially violent situations. Reactive management strategies also need to be worked out with staff on a very individual basis, taking into account client behaviour and staff skills and competencies.

The legacy of behaviour modification means that staff do sometimes perceive such strategies as treatment, whereas in fact the 'treatment' is a combination of designing the environment, of designing individual programmes, and designing specific ways of developing more appropriate behaviour.

Risk-taking

Inevitably when working with individuals who present challenges, there are risks. These risks may be of injury to others (including the general public, other clients, staff, family members), injury to the client themselves, damage to property and the like. A clear analysis of the risk, its likelihood of occurring, its consequences, ways of reducing it and an agreed judgement as to how important it is to take the risk needs to be undertaken (see **Module Nine**).

References

Department of Health (1993) *Services for People with Learning Disabilities and Challenging Behaviour or Mental Health Needs: Report of a Project Group (Chair: Professor J. L. Mansell).* London: Department of Health.

Emerson, E., Barrett, S., Bell, C., Cummings, R., McCool, C. & Toogood, A. (1987) *Developing Services for People with Severe Learning Difficulties and Challenging Behaviours.* Canterbury: Institute of Social and Applied Psychology, University of Kent.

Felce, D. & Lowe, K. (1993) Supporting people with severe learning difficulties and challenging behaviour in ordinary housing. In: C. Kierman (Ed.) *Research to Practice? Implications of research on the challenging behaviour of people with learning disability.* British Institute of Learning Disabilities Publications, Frankfurt Lodge, Clevedon Hall, Victoria Road, Clevedon, Avon BS21 7SJ.

80

Iwata, B., Dorsey, M., Slifer, K., Bauman, K. & Richman, G. (1982) Towards a functional analysis of self-injury. *Analysis and Intervention in Developmental Disabilities,* **2**, 3–20.

King, T. M. (1995) *Reactive Management Strategies.* London: Lewisham and Guy's Mental Health NHS Trust.

McGill, P. & Toogood, A. (1994) Providing helpful environments. In: E. Emerson, P. McGill & J. Mansell (Eds.) *Severe Learning Disabilities and Challenging Behaviours – Designing high quality services.* London: Chapman and Hall.

Murphy, G. (1994) Understanding challenging behaviour. In: E. Emerson, P. McGill & J. Mansell (Eds.) *Severe Learning Disabilities and Challenging Behaviours – Designing high quality services.* London: Chapman and Hall.

Sinason, V. (1992) *Mental Handicap and the Human Condition: New approaches from the Tavistock.* London: Free Association Books.

Slater, E. & Roth, M. (1969) Mental subnormality. *Clinical Psychiatry,* 692–735. London: Bailliere, Tindall and Cassell.

Turk, V. & Brown, H. (1993) Sexual abuse of adults with a learning disability: Results of a two-year incidence survey. *Mental Handicap Research,* **6**, 193–216.

Willis, T., La Vigna, G. & Donnellan, A. (1987) *Behaviour Assessment Guide.* California: Institute for Applied Behavior Analysis.

Willis, T. & La Vigna, G. (1985) *Reinforcement Inventory for Adults.* California: Institute for Applied Behavior Analysis.

MENTAL HEALTH SERVICE FACTORS

Geraldine Holt and Nick Bouras

Over recent years there has been a phasing out of mental handicap hospitals in the UK, with a reduction of 26,000 beds between 1980 and 1993 (Emerson & Hatton, 1994). This process continues. The nature of the services developed in the community to replace this provision has varied. There has been a recognition that people with learning disabilities who are mentally ill, have behaviour problems or offend, require a range of specialist facilities and services (Department of Health, 1989). However, most policies have focused on meeting educational and social care needs rather than mental health needs. The *Mansell Report* (DoH, 1993) sought to address this issue and proposed guidelines for commissioners of services and a charter for people with learning disabilities who have challenging behaviour or mental health needs. More recently the *Health of the Nation* initiative included a strategy to reduce ill-health and death caused by mental illness in those with learning disabilities (DoH, 1995).

Services developed to meet the mental health needs of people with learning disabilities

Residential services

In this model, in-patient and out-patient facilities are often concentrated within a **hospital** setting with the added possibility of outreach work.

The suggested advantages of this approach include:

- the creation of a secure and controlled environment

- the provision of a comprehensive range of services

- the development of staff expertise

83

- the economic use of specialist staff time, including high levels of nursing staff support

- sharing of on-site occupational training and recreational facilities for clients

- provision of asylum for those who need it

- the minimisation of disruption to other service users.

This model questions the ability of small local units to cope with severely disturbed people and suggests possible difficulties in arranging medical cover and staff support (Day, 1994).

One difficulty with such units is linking meaningfully with the client's friends, family and local services, which are sometimes a distance away. This is particularly relevant when the mental health needs are caused by challenging behaviour rather than mental illness where the continuity of approach is vital; for example, the preliminary evaluation of one such service suggested some success in the assessment and functional analyses carried out within the unit, but less success in the management of specific behavioural problems in the long term (Murphy *et al.*, 1991). This is possibly due to the fact that the implementation of the recommended care plans depends on the agreement of the local services to which the client is discharged, as well as their competency and facilities to apply the required techniques. Furthermore, continuing support and clinical involvement from professionals specialising in this area following discharge is needed; something frequently lacking.

Non-residential services

In this model, specialist services provide their input in the **community**. Such services may be linked with learning disabilities services, but integration with generic mental health services may be difficult (Bicknell 1985), or be linked with generic mental health services. This latter is the model in which the authors work and will be described in more detail.

Community specialist psychiatric services (CSPS) integrated with the generic mental health and learning disabilities service

In this particular model, the specialist psychiatric service for people with learning disabilities becomes part of the mainstream mental health service, and can use all of its facilities, including acute and medium-stay in-patient beds and a variety of community resources. Unnecessary duplication is therefore avoided (Bouras *et al.*, 1994). This model has been developed in south-east London following the resettlement of people with learning disabilities from a long-stay institution and the closure of all long-stay hospitals in the area.

Figure 1 below outlines the essential components of the Community Specialist Psychiatric Service in routine practice.

Figure 1   Essential Components of the Community Specialist Psychiatric Service

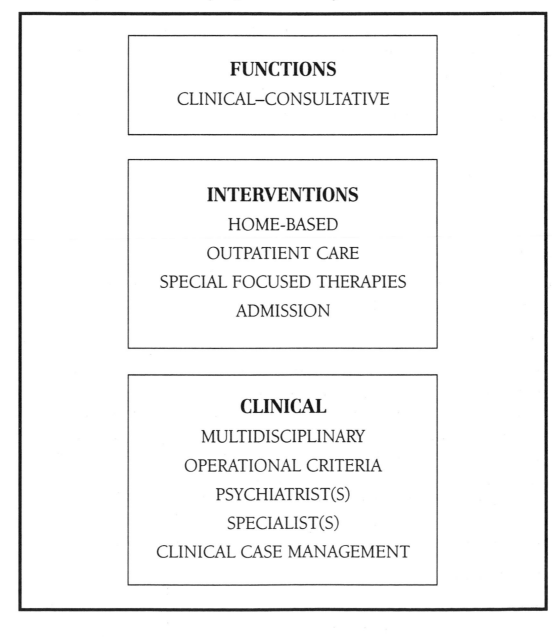

FUNCTIONS
CLINICAL–CONSULTATIVE

INTERVENTIONS
HOME-BASED
OUTPATIENT CARE
SPECIAL FOCUSED THERAPIES
ADMISSION

CLINICAL
MULTIDISCIPLINARY
OPERATIONAL CRITERIA
PSYCHIATRIST(S)
SPECIALIST(S)
CLINICAL CASE MANAGEMENT

85

Functions

The CSPS has two broad functions: **clinical** and **service-related**.

The **clinical components** of the CSPS include: psychiatric assessment and treatment of adults with psychiatric disorders; management of behavioural problems; work with offenders, including the interface with the courts; and the management of the psychological impact of chronic disabilities, including epilepsy.

All referrals receive a detailed assessment and are presented and discussed at weekly community clinical meetings, where a therapeutic intervention plan is formulated.

The **service-related** roles include regular consultation and support to multi-disciplinary community teams, social services, voluntary and private organisations, day centres, service managers, relatives and care staff. Through this role, complex care programmes are supervised and a multiplier effect is achieved on a larger number of staff and clients. Assistance with accessing and making links with the community support network is also offered.

Participation in training initiatives, particulaly skills transfer to care staff, and the generation of ideas for improving and developing the service are also parts of this service's role.

Interventions

A range of therapeutic methods can be used, depending on clients' needs. These methods can be applied in different settings.

Home-based

This is the preferred intervention, as it occurs in the client's normal environment and focuses where the identified behaviour is occurring. Thus, it directly involves the people with whom the client interacts as important agents for producing and maintaining change. The nature and frequency of staff contacts are determined by each client's individual needs. An individual care plan is usually devised following the initial assessment, which may involve more than one visit. Objectives of the intervention are identified and agreed with the client, wherever possible, and his or her carers. Behaviour-modification principles and pharmacotherapy are commonly used. Services are provided indefinitely, permitting long-term continuity of care.

Out-patient care

Clients attend regular out-patient clinics based in general hospitals for assessment, review of their care plan and monitoring of their medication. Attendance at out-patient clinics is particularly useful for organising various clinical and laboratory tests for clients as well as liaising with medical services.

Special focused therapies

These include psychotherapy (individual and group), social skills training and psychosexual counselling, and are provided on an out-patient basis.

Admission to **psychiatric units** occurs when necessary. Acute psychiatric beds are available in a designated generic psychiatric ward, but the clinical care of the admitted client is taken over by the specialist psychiatric service in learning disabilities, in liaison with the ward nursing staff.

Clinical team

The clinical team works out clear operational criteria of the clients who can access the specialist service.

The clinical team referred to in this text consists of consultant psychiatrists, psychiatrists in training and community psychiatric nurses with expertise in both learning disabilities and mental health. Input by clinical psychologists is received through the multidisciplinary mainstream learning disabilities services. It is important to examine some of the weaknesses of this approach which could be described as system problems and service delivery problems.

Problems

System problems

These problems are mainly political, administrative, bureaucratic, ideological and philosophical. They are related to funding issues and available resources, professional rivalries and unclear operational policies.

Service-delivery problems

These include the lack of in-patient treatment for people with severe learning disabilities, whose needs cannot be met in acute psychiatric wards. There is also a shortage of medium-term residential treatment for stabilisation, as well as a shortage of facilities for people who offend, and for the elderly.

Conclusions

The implementation of the new community care legislation has shifted the emphasis of care for people with learning disabilities to local authorities. One of the main challenges facing multiprofessional teams will be how to avoid the situation of cost rather than quality becoming the crucial service-delivery issue. The operation of a coherent specialist team model, focused on a defined population of people with learning disabilities and mental health needs, including psychiatric disorders, will, it is hoped, avoid the fragmentation and confusions associated with rapidly changing external service environments.

References and further reading

Bicknell, J. (1985) The mental handicap service. In: D. Sines & J. Bicknell (Eds.) *Caring for Mentally Handicapped People in the Community*. London: Harper and Row. 9–37.

Bouras, N., Brooks, D. & Drummond, K. (1994) Community psychiatric services for people with mental retardation. In: N. Bouras (Ed.) *Mental Health in Mental Retardation*. Cambridge: Cambridge University Press.

Day, K. (1994) Psychiatric services in mental retardation: Generic or specialised provision? In: N. Bouras, (Ed.) *Mental Health in Mental Retardation*. Cambridge: Cambridge University Press.

Department of Health (1989) *Needs and Responses: Services for adults with mental handicap who are mentally ill, who have behaviour problems or who offend*. London: HMSO. ISBN 1 85197 431 8.

Department of Health (1993) *Services for people with learning disabilities and challenging behaviour or mental health needs*. Chairman: Professor J. L. Mansell. London: HMSO.

Department of Health (1995) *The Health of the Nation: A strategy for people with learning disabilities*. London: HMSO.

Emerson, E. & Hatton, C. (1994) *Moving Out: Relocation from hospital to community*. London: HMSO.

Murphy, G., Holland, A., Fowler, P. & Repp, J. (1991) MIETS: A service option for people with mild mental handicaps and challenging behaviour or psychiatric problems. *Mental Handicap Research,* **4** (1) 41–66.

THE AETIOLOGY OF
LEARNING DISABILITIES

Sarah H. Bernard

The aetiology, or cause, of a person's learning disabilities is important for a number of reasons. These include:

- the need for the parents, carers and individuals to understand why learning disabilities have occurred

- possible treatment of specific conditions

- identification of complications of the disorder

- understanding of how the disorder may develop over time

- risks to other family members of the condition re-occurring in their offspring.

Classification

The causes of learning disabilities may be divided into **genetic** and **environmental**, although these categories may overlap (Russell, 1985). In general, genetic causes originate prior to conception or during the very early development of the fetus. Environmental causes include those that effect the developing fetus or those that occur in the perinatal, neonatal or childhood period.

Another way of classifying the causes of learning disabilities is to identify the **stage of development** that the disorder originated from; for example:

- prefertilisation

- intrauterine

- perinatal

- postnatal

- unknown.

Table 5 The Aetiology of Learning Disabilities

STAGE OF DEVELOPMENT	ABNORMALITY		EXAMPLES
PREFERTILISATION	CHROMOSOMAL		
	Autosome	trisomy monosomy triploidy translocation deletion	Down syndrome Turner's syndrome *Cri-du-chat* syndrome
	Sex chromosome		Fragile-X syndrome
	MONOGENIC	dominant recessive sex-linked	tuberous sclerosis phenylketonuria Lesch-Nyhan
	MULTIFACTORIAL	central nervous system malformations	spina bifida
INTRAUTERINE	INFECTIONS	viral other	cytomegalic inclusion virus (CMV)/ rubella/HIV toxoplasmosis
	DIET	deficiencies	neural tube defect
	TOXINS	alcohol smoking	
	MATERNAL DISEASE	pre-eclampsia thyroid diabetes	sacral agenesis
	PHYSICAL	trauma radiation	amniotic bands
PERINATAL	ABNORMAL GROWTH	prematurity intrauterine growth retardation	
	TRAUMA	twins obstructed birth instrumental birth	breech
POSTNATAL	INFECTION	bacterial viral	meningitis herpes
	TOXINS	lead carbon monoxide vaccine	
	PHYSICAL	non-accidental injury road traffic accident deprivation	

Prefertilisation causes include those that are of a genetic origin: chromosomal abnormalities and single gene defects. Examples include Down syndrome and Fragile-X.

Intrauterine causes may be due to infection, toxins, maternal diet, maternal disease or trauma. An example is rubella infection.

Perinatal causes are those occurring around the time of delivery and include trauma, hypoxia, prematurity and growth retardation. Trauma may occur in complicated deliveries.

Finally, **postnatal** causes include infection, toxins and trauma; for example, meningitis is one infection that can cause learning disabilities.

Table 5 opposite gives further examples of these causes.

When diagnosing the cause of an individual's learning disabilities, it is important that the correct diagnosis is made. Generally, the paediatrician and clinical geneticist will be involved with this. The child and parents will be offered detailed counselling and tests to elucidate the cause where possible.

Common syndromes associated with learning disabilities

There has always been an interest in people who appear different to the norm. Historically, 'freaks' and 'monsters' were exhibited in circuses and shows. In our society, we have advanced to a stage where it is recognised that certain people, although individuals, have a number of features in common with each other but different to the majority of the population, i.e. a syndrome.

There are many syndromes associated with learning disabilities; refer to a major text for further information (such as McKuisick, 1988).

The interest in specific syndromes in learning disabilities has become topical as it is recognised that, apart from similarities in physical features, there are identifiable behaviours that occur more commonly in certain syndromes.

Examples of these are:

● Down syndrome

● Fragile-X syndrome

● Prader-Willi syndrome

- Lesch-Nyhan syndrome

- tuberous sclerosis.

In this chapter, we concentrate on two of the most common causes of learning disabilities (Turk, 1994): **Down syndrome** and **Fragile-X syndrome**. Details are summarised in **Tables 6** and **7** on pages 93 and 94.

Down syndrome

Down syndrome is one of the more common chromosomal anomalies associated with learning disabilities. The overall incidence is approximately one-in-700 live births, although a further 50% result in a spontaneous abortion and 20% are stillborn. Incidence increases with maternal age, so at 20 years of age a mother has a one-in-1,500 chance of delivering a child with Down syndrome. This goes up to a one-in-50 chance at 43 years of age. Prenatal screening and diagnosis may be offered.

People with Down syndrome have a characteristic appearance with up-slanting eyes, Brushfield spots (speckles in the iris), a small nose and a rather flat face. The infant might be hypotonic and have low-set ears. A Simian crease (single palmar crease) may be present in 50% of those affected with the syndrome.

People with Down syndrome have associated learning disabilities. They are also at risk from congenital heart abnormalities, cataracts, epilepsy, thyroid disorder and leukaemia.

In Down syndrome, 95% of cases are due to an extra chromosome 21 (trisomy 21). Some four per cent of cases are as a result of a translocation and a further one per cent are due to mosaicism.

People with Down syndrome are at risk of developing dementia later in life (Connor & Ferguson-Smith, 1993).

Fragile-X syndrome

This occurs when there is an abnormal area on one of the X chromosomes. Men and women can be affected, although more frequently females are carriers and pass the abnormal chromosome onto their male offspring. It is possible for the diagnosis to be made in pregnancy, and carrier women can also be detected.

The incidence of Fragile-X syndrome is probably one in 1,000, with five per cent of males having severe learning disabilities, but 20% of males being unaffected. Around 30% of carrier females are affected by the syndrome.

Table 6 Down syndrome

SYNDROME	DOWN SYNDROME
OTHER NAMES	Mongol (no longer used)
GENETICS	Trisomy 21 5% translocations 1% mozaics
SCREENING/DIAGNOSIS	Bart's test chorionic villus sampling amniocentesis karyotyping
EPIDEMIOLOGY	1/700 live births maternal age-related more common in males
FEATURES	low birth weight hypotonic upslanting palpabral fissures Brushfield spots flat occiput epicanthic folds low-set ears small mouth flat nasal bridge short fifth finger Simian crease congenital heart disease cataracts hypothyroid leukaemia sensory problems
PSYCHIATRIC/BEHAVIOURAL PROBLEMS	dementia stereotyped behaviour
OTHER	stigma family problems

Table 7 Fragile-X syndrome

SYNDROME	FRAGILE-X SYNDROME
OTHER NAMES	Martin Bell syndrome
GENETICS	Fragile site distal end of long arm of X chromosome – position Xq27.3 Failure of normal chromatid condensation in mitosis
SCREENING/DIAGNOSIS	Direct DNA analysis now possible Culture in folate-deficient media
EPIDEMIOLOGY	1/1000 in general population 5% males with severe learning disabilities 20% males unaffected 30% carrier females with the Fragile-X site are affected
FEATURES	joint laxity long face large ears macro-orchidism cardiac abnormalities dysplasia soft skin large head long nose
PSYCHIATRIC/BEHAVIOURAL	autistic features hyperactivity
OTHER	cognitive deficits speech abnormalities

The physical features of the Fragile-X syndrome are quite variable and cannot be used to make a diagnosis. People with it have lax joints, a long face and large ears, large testicles, cardiac abnormalities and a large head with a long nose. A number of behaviours are associated with Fragile-X syndrome, including autistic-type behaviours and hyperactivity. People with it also have specific cognitive deficits and speech abnormalities (Turk, 1994).

Prevention of learning disabilities

The causes of learning disabilities have previously been described as occurring prefertilisation, intrauterine, perinatally and postnatally. This framework is also of use when considering methods of prevention of learning disabilities.

In general, the prefertilisation causes of learning disabilities are genetic in origin. Primary prevention can only be achieved by genetic manipulation and this is currently in its experimental stages. Secondary prevention is possible with the use of termination of pregnancy. There are obvious ethical, legal and religious factors complicating this preventative method. The *1990 Abortion Act* permits termination up to 24 weeks' gestation although, in certain rare cases, it may occur later in the pregnancy.

Intrauterine causes of learning disabilities may be prevented by improved obstetric care, as may perinatal causes.

Postnatally, learning disabilities may be prevented by detection of treatable causes, improved social conditions and road safety.

References and further reading

McKuisick, V. A. (1988) *Mendelian Inheritance in Man*, 8th Edition. Baltimore: John Hopkins University Press.

Russell, O. (1985) *Mental Handicap*. Edinburgh: Churchill Livingstone Publications.

Turk, J. (1994) The Fragile-X syndrome. In: N. Bouras (Ed.) *Mental Health in Mental Retardation*. Cambridge University Press.

Connor, J. M. & Ferguson-Smith, M. A. (1993) *Essential Medical Genetics*. Oxford: Blackwell Scientific Publications.

95

EPILEPSY IN PEOPLE WITH LEARNING DISABILITIES

David Brooks

There is a strong relationship between severe brain damage, severe learning disabilities and epilepsy. The prevalence of epilepsy in people with severe learning disabilities is 30%, and in people with profound learning disabilities 50%. In contrast, the prevalence for people with mild learning disabilities is six per cent (Rutter *et al.*, 1970).

People with learning disabilities are susceptible to all forms of epilepsy. Sometimes epilepsy and learning disabilities are both consequences of brain damage. For example, there is a high association between epilepsy and disorders such as cerebral palsy and tuberous sclerosis.

People with Down syndrome now have an increased life span and epilepsy is being diagnosed more frequently. Recent studies have shown that the incidence of epilepsy increases with age. It seems likely that this may be linked to the Alzheimer-like changes seen in such individuals.

Assessment

Assessment of the individual must be comprehensive and encompass social and environmental factors as well as medical. Monitoring of epilepsy begins with a sound base-line of factual information regarding the nature of the epilepsy, its causes and associations. Seizure charts must also record ongoing events. See **Table 8** overleaf.

Making the diagnosis of epilepsy has important implications for the functioning and lifestyle of the individual. Hence the diagnosis must be soundly justified.

The diagnosis of epilepsy in people with learning disabilities can be extremely difficult. The person may be unable to give a clear account of their symptoms.

97

Table 8 Assessment and Management Checklist

Base-line

1. Cause of learning disabilities

    . . . .

2. Adaptive functioning, skills, psychometric testing, methods of communication, developmental level

    . . . .

3. Personality factors, attitudes, beliefs, health, concepts, coping strategies

    . . . .

4. Past and present medical history and relevant treatments

    . . . .

5. Past and present psychiatric history and relevant treatments

    . . . .

    . . . .

    . . . .

    . . . .

6. Special sensory problems

    . . . .

7. Special medical considerations

    . . . .

8. Past and present behaviour problems

    . . . .

9. Relevant investigations

    . . . .

10. Psychosocial factors, psychosexual factors

    . . . .

11. Lifestyle and interest

    . . . .

12. Ethical and cultural issues

    . . . .

98

Epilepsy

1. Cause

2. Onset . . . .

3. Type . . . .

4. Frequency . . . .

5. Relevant investigations

    . . . .

6. Changes in base-line factors

    . . . .

7. Associations   ● Reflex epilepsy. . . . .

                      ● Drug interactions. . . . .

                      ● Menstrual cycle/menarche . . . .

                      ● Stress . . . .

                      ● Other (psychosocial factors, life events, medical
    and psychiatric disorders) . . . .

8. Treatment   ● Drugs . . . .

                      ● Efficacy/compliance. . . . .

                      ● Monitoring procedures. . . . .

                      ● Relevant ongoing investigations . . . .

                      ● Side-effects and drug interactions. . . . .

                      ● Behavioural therapies. . . . .

                      ● Psychological therapies . . . .

                      ● Social interventions . . . .

                      ● Treatment of other medical and
    psychiatric disorders . . . .

                      ● Health education. . . . .

9. Risk assessment

    . . . .

    Medication policy

    . . . .

    Service access

    . . . .

Psychometric testing and sophisticated investigation may not be possible or practical. Getting to know the individual, speaking to informants, and being familiar with the person's past medical history and psychosocial functioning will be important tools in diagnosis.

It can be difficult to differentiate epilepsy from non-epileptic behaviour. Aggression, bizarre behaviour, abnormal motor activity, neurological deficits, the side-effects of drugs, self-injurious behaviour and generalised poor response to the environment may all be part of the repertoire of a person with learning disabilities without the presence of epilepsy. However, such features may be present alongside epilepsy. A detailed account by an observer of the suspect behaviour is invaluable in making a diagnosis.

People with learning disabilities may also have physical disabilities. There is also a strong positive association between emotional disorders and epilepsy. Studies of children with epilepsy in the general population show that 25% have significant psychiatric disorders. School-age children with complicated epilepsy who are in institutions show 70% with significant psychiatric disorders (Corbett & Trimble, 1983). Aggression is, however, rarely associated with the epileptic attack itself. People may feel stigmatised and have low self-esteem. To suffer from epilepsy as well may exacerbate their negative self-image and cause psychological problems.

Management

Psychosocial

People with learning disabilities and epilepsy often experience difficulties in psychosocial functioning, particularly in the field of inter-personal relationships.

Such difficulties may present to the physician only in the form of poorly-controlled seizures, non-compliance with medication, or changes in behaviour and symptom patterns. The impact of epilepsy, as well as learning disabilities and mental health needs, can produce major difficulties with relationships. It is important to support and counsel individuals to help them and their carers to accept the disorder. This must be done in the context of issues of consent, health education, and an understanding of the individual's values, concepts of illness, abilities and developmental level. They must understand and cope with the real limitations imposed by epilepsy. The individual may resist this by denying the presence of the disorder, or may put all the responsibility on family and carers. Family or house dynamics may reinforce this. It is important to provide a physical environment that is safe but conducive to self-development and independence. This will include assessment of risk in areas such as activities and self-administration of medication.

Psychological treatment has implications for improving seizure control and possibly reducing medication. In addition, behavioural techniques, including bio-feedback and relaxation, have been shown to be of value.

People with epilepsy and learning disabilities face an added problem of restricted job and educational opportunities because of their seizures. Psychiatric and behaviour disorders associated with epilepsy may create employment difficulties and reinforce the psychological difficulties that the person has. Another contributory factor is the negative attitudes of others. Studies have shown that 25–75% of people with epilepsy have vocational problems. Organisations must foster appropriate attitudes to epilepsy.

There are imaginative work schemes for people with learning disabilities to help integrate them into useful employment. Advocates can be of value in terms of recruitment and counselling. There has been active campaigning from Scope, The Royal Association for Disability and Rehabilitation and other organisations to improve employment opportunities. Social skills training is important for people with psychosocial and cognitive deficits (Edwards *et al.*, 1986).

Medical

The basic principles of epilepsy treatment are the same as for people without learning disabilities. However, we are dealing with more severe and mixed types of seizures and the frequency of seizures is usually higher. This may result in the use of more than one medicine with increased side-effects. However, the vast majority of such people do obtain seizure control on one medicine. There is also evidence that the effectiveness of medicines is probably less in people with extensive brain damage.

Barbiturates are discouraged for use in people with learning disabilities, particularly children and the elderly, because of their sedative and addictive effects. Carbamazepine is a popular and useful drug, as it not only treats the seizures but may help to control emotional problems.

The issue of combined anti-epileptic medication and psychotropic medication is controversial and a difficult clinical problem, as neuroleptics and most anti-depressants lower the seizure threshold. However, it may be necessary to treat a psychiatric disorder or help control behaviour, and the dose of anticonvulsant may have to be increased to compensate for this.

Because of the difficulty in seizure management and in diagnosing side-effects, monitoring of blood levels may be useful.

It is important to strive for the use of one medicine at the lowest effective dose. Ideally the medicine with the lowest toxicity should be used. It is also important not to be too conservative in the medical management of people with learning disabilities and epilepsy, in order that they might benefit from new developments and medicines.

In addition to physically dangerous side-effects, including effects on intellectual functioning, one must bear in mind the more subtle social effects of medication — such as hairiness, obesity, gum swelling and coarsening of facial features — which will further stigmatise the individual and provide even greater social rejection. Medication is further discussed in **Chapter VII**.

Adequate staff training to recognise epilepsy and its associations, both medical and psychosocial, is vital. This will also be important in creating a more effective working relationship between carers, doctors and other professionals (Oxley & Smith, 1991).

Services

With good co-ordination between the family/carers, GPs, hospital and local authority services, the vast majority of people with learning disabilities and epilepsy can have a high standard of care in the community, based on a multidisciplinary approach.

Various reports have recommended the establishment of special epilepsy clinics at a district general hospital level, and the development of regional neurological and research centres attached to appropriate departments of neurology, psychiatry and paediatrics.

Residential units might also be provided, to allow assessment and supervision under ordinary living and working conditions (DHSS, 1986). Residential schools also exist which cater specifically for children with epilepsy.

The community team for people with learning disabilities and the psychiatrist are useful resources for treatment, medical advocacy and liaison with other relevant services. Because of the increased responsibilities of general practitioners and primary care teams in meeting the medical and social needs of people with learning disabilities and epilepsy, adequate training and a good working relationship with members of the multidisciplinary team and other medical disciplines are essential.

Conclusion

The prevention, early diagnosis and treatment of epilepsy is essential to avoid additional handicaps for people with learning disabilities. Not only the seizures themselves but also their treatment may affect cognition, behaviour and the person's psychosocial life. As with so many other care and treatment issues for people with learning disabilities, the key to the management of epilepsy is to achieve a balance between allowing individual freedom and risk-taking, and protecting and promoting the health of the individual.

References

Corbett, J. A. & Trimble, M. R. (1983) Epilepsy and anticonvulsant medication. In: M. Rutter (Ed.) *Developmental Neuropsychiatry*. New York: Guildford Press.

DHSS (1986) *Health Service Development Services for People with Epilepsy*. London: HMSO.

Edwards, F., Espir, M. & Oxley, J. (Eds.) (1986) *Epilepsy Employment*. RSM Services, No. 86. London: Royal Society of Medicine.

Oxley & Smith (1991) *The Epilepsy Reference Book*. London: Faber & Faber.

Rutter, M., Graham, P. & Yule, W. (1970) A Neuropsychiatric Study in Childhood Clinics. In: *Developmental Medicine*, 35–36. London: Heinemann.

103

STRESS AND BURNOUT

Geraldine Holt and Barley Oliver

What is stress?

Stress can be defined in many ways. It results from an interaction between a person and his or her environment. Menaghan and Merves (1984) defined stress as a *'discrepancy between environmental demands and individual capabilities'*.

Sources of stress

It is clear from the definition above that stress results from the interplay of a number of factors. Hatton and Emerson (1993) summarise these potential sources of stress as:

● within the person; for example, personality factors, health

● within the clients with whom the member of staff is working; for example, challenging behaviours, level of intellectual disability

● within the organisation where the person works; for example, level of support, work overload, job variety, income, role conflict.

Whilst all of these factors are important, the research in this area points to organisational characteristics of the person's work as being most commonly reported as contributing to perceived stress. For example, Hatton and Emerson (1993) collected questionnaire data from 64 direct-care staff in a residential facility for people with multiple disabilities. Here, staff stress was related to support from other staff, job variety, their perception of organisational democracy, goodness-of-fit between the attitudes of staff and management, opportunities for development and income. These results are echoed by those of other workers. Social support between direct care staff and between direct care staff and their immediate supervisor is important in reducing stress. Rose (1995), in a review of the literature, suggests social support is important as a buffer against stressors that effect physical and mental health. He states: 'It is possible that social contact with co-workers, immediate manager and residents can become progressively more important with greater geographical isolation in smaller community facilities.' This is obviously a crucial factor to consider in planning services now that they are so dispersed in small staffed houses in the community.

Another emerging factor is the coping strategies employed by staff (Hatton *et al.*, 1995). The evidence seems to be that some staff use 'wishful thinking strategies' as opposed to 'practical coping strategies'. Staff who employ wishful thinking strategies seem to experience greater levels of stress. Practical coping strategies are represented by staff who choose statements like: 'I try to analyse the situation in order to understand it better', as opposed to staff who choose wishful thinking statements like: 'I wish the situation would go away or somehow be over with.'

Ward (1989) also demonstrated the importance of issues related to clients. She interviewed residential staff in two supported houses for adults with learning disabilities. In addition to the organisational factors highlighted above, other key factors which emerged were: coping with some people's aggression and mental problems, and difficulties in helping people learn new skills.

Kroese and Fleming (1992) interestingly report that whilst care staff in their study found teaching clients and accompanying them on outings stressful, these were also important areas of considerable job satisfaction.

Results of stress

As the Kroese and Fleming study illustrates, the result of stress is not necessarily negative. Where stress is satisfactorily coped with, it can lead to a sense of achievement and personal development. However, stress is often experienced as negative and overwhelming.

The response of the individual can be divided into four categories:

- **physical**; for example, feeling tired, coronary heart disease

- **emotional**; for example, irritability, mental health needs

- **cognitive**; for example, poor concentration, poor memory

- **behavioural**; for example, alcohol abuse, poor eating habits.

Prolonged stress may lead to burnout:

> '*emotional exhaustion and cynicism that occurs frequently among individuals who do "people-work" of some kind*'
>
> (Maslach, 1982).

Maslach described three main features of this syndrome:

● emotional exhaustion (tiredness, somatic symptoms, irritability, accident-proneness, depression and excessive alcohol consumption)

● depersonalisation (treating clients and other people as if they are objects, clients are viewed as bringing their difficulties on themselves)

● low sense of personal accomplishment.

Burnout has been reported among both direct-care and supervisory staff in residential facilities for people with learning disabilities. Firth *et al.* (1986) present evidence to suggest that nurses who report feelings of depersonalisation show less respect to their subordinates. Knapp *et al.* (1989), reporting on 28 community care projects, found that for 21% of staff leaving the projects, their departure was attributable to stress, dissatisfaction or conflict. The effects of stress, therefore, are important not only for the individual, but also for those around the person: family, friends, colleagues and clients.

Individual ways of coping with stress

Wycherley (1990) suggests the following framework to address stress:

● **Look after yourself**
For example: eat a sensible diet, take adequate rest and regular exercise, develop and use a support network.

● **Knowing yourself and what you want**
For example: recognise potential sources of strain and plan for these, acknowledge and express feelings, take responsibility for your own life.

● **Manage work**
For example: set priorities, say 'no', delegate, take breaks.

● **Develop skills**
For example: plan use of time, reward success, reward others.

Whilst each individual should take responsibility for coping personally with stress, for this to be effective, such effort needs to be supported by the systems around the person, so that he or she is working with these systems rather than against them.

Organisational ways of reducing stress

In staffed houses, organisational issues to reduce stress need to be given a priority to try and counteract the stressors already highlighted, such as staff isolation and role ambiguity. The service needs to be structured so that teamwork can meaningfully develop, staff can be clear about what is expected of them and whether they are achieving this. It is also important that they feel there is a framework of support around them. Bearing all these factors in mind, the following elements of service organisation are suggested as vital:

- **Constructive supervision** is very helpful to staff. It needs to be given a high priority by management. Staff need to know they will receive regular supervision; when they will be helped to identify what they are doing right; identify clear, achievable tasks; and be supported in areas they find emotionally or practically difficult. This should have lots of positive outcomes, including helping staff to move away from 'wishful thinking' strategies.

- There is a need to have in place a system of staff support for when things go wrong. A **debriefing procedure** so that staff are not left to cope with the after-effects of, for example, being attacked and possibly injured by a client. Staff need support in order to avoid feeling to blame for things that have happened, and to receive help in resolving some of the emotions they are left with like fear and anger.

- To increase team work and staff being able to influence the service, **regular staff meetings** where important issues are discussed and actions agreed are seen as a necessary part of any service.

- To clarify staff roles and to ensure staff and clients can celebrate achievements, an **individual planning system** should be in place with a clear key worker system identified.

- For staff working with clients who present a challenge to services through their behaviour, it is often important to have **risk assessments** developed which state the type of risks involved, what the degree of risk is, what actions are to be taken to minimise the risks, and what staff should do if the worst scenario occurs. It is vital that these assessments are agreed by a group of staff to show the decisions have been taken carefully, and responsibility is shared. Management guidelines are also needed at times so that staff have an agreed way to consistently respond to a client's difficult behaviours.

108

Conclusion

In order for staff to be able to enjoy the rewards of working in this area, they must be able to cope with co-existent stress positively. This will improve job satisfaction and reduce staff turnover — both positive features — not only for the clients but also for the organisation.

By addressing the issues raised in this chapter, it is hoped that individuals and staff groups will be enabled to cope with stress positively.

References and further reading

Firth, H., McIntee, J., McKeown, P. & Britton, P. (1986) Interpersonal support among nurses at work. *Journal of Advanced Nursing,* **11**, 273–282.

Hatton, C., Brown, R., Caine, E. & Emerson, E. (1995) Stressors, coping strategies and stress-related outcomes among direct care staff in staffed houses for people with learning disabilities. *Mental Handicap Research,* **8**, (4), 252–271.

Hatton, C. & Emerson, E. (1993) Organisational predictors of staff stress, satisfaction, and intended turnover in a service for people with multiple disabilities. *Mental Retardation,* **31**, (6), 388–395.

Knapp, M., Cambridge, P. & Thornason, C. (1989) *Final Report of an Evaluation of the Care in the Community Initiative.* Canterbury: Personal Social Services Research Unit, University of Kent.

Kroese, B. S. & Fleming, I. (1992) Staff's attitudes and working conditions in community-based group homes of people with mental handicap. *Mental Handicap Research,* **5**, (1), 82–101.

Maslach, C. (1982) *Burnout – The cost of caring.* New York: Prentice Hall Press.

Menaghan, E. G. & Merves, E. S. (1984) Coping with occupational problems: The limits of individual efforts. *Journal of Health and Social Behaviour,* **25** (Dec.), 406–423.

Rose, J. (1995) Stress and residential staff: towards an integration of existing research. *Mental Handicap Research,* **8**, (4), 220–236.

Ward, L. (1989) An ordinary life: the early views and experiences of residential staff in the Wells Road Service. *Mental Handicap,* **17**, 6–9.

Wycherley, R. J. (1990) *Stress at Work.* St Leonards on Sea: Outset Publishing Ltd.

109

LEGAL AND ETHICAL ISSUES

John Gavilan and Andrea Hughes

This chapter deals with the legal and ethical issues in relation to learning disabilities and mental health needs. It is divided into the following sections:

1   General overview and explanation of the *Mental Health Act 1983*

2   Specific sections of the *Mental Health Act 1983*

3   *Mental Health (Patients in the Community) Act 1995*

4   Consent

5   Risk taking

6   Ethical issues

General overview and explanation of the Mental Health Act 1983

Overview

People with learning disabilities have the same rights and responsibilities as everyone else. As minors, their parents can exercise certain rights on their behalf. As adults — i.e. when they reach eighteen, and in some cases from sixteen — those parental rights cease.

Whilst much of the law relating to people with learning disabilities is general law which applies to everyone, or has been adopted from general principles of law to cover learning disabilities, there are instances when the need for specific legislation has been recognised.

Problems arise for people with learning disabilities, not because they do not have rights, but because they may not have the ability to express or exercise those rights, or because others may be disinclined to recognise those rights.

Explanation of the Mental Health Act 1983

The *Mental Health Act 1983* regulates the care of 'mentally abnormal persons'. Parts IV and V of the Act provide a legal basis for compulsory admission and detention of psychiatric patients.

Under the Act, there are three main groups of compulsory orders for assessment and treatment:

(i)   Assessment orders (Sections 2, 4, 5 (2), 135 and 136)

(ii)   Treatment orders (Sections 3 and 7)

(iii)   Admission and transfer of patients concerned with criminal proceedings (Sections 37/ 41, 47 and 49).

The **short-term** orders listed in (i) apply to any **mental disorder** which **need not be specified**. For the long-term orders listed in (ii) and (iii), it must be stated that the patient suffers from one of the four types of mental disorders:

(i)   Mental illness

(ii)   Severe mental impairment

(iii)   Mental impairment

(iv)   Psychopathic disorder.

The *Mental Health Act* does not define mental illness but leaves this as a matter of clinical judgement, although it does provide guidelines. The other three types of mental disorder are defined.

People with learning disabilities do not *automatically* fit into the category of mental impairment.

Thus, when considering using the *Mental Health Act* for compulsory admission for people with learning disabilities, it is important to distinguish between the terms *'learning disabilities'* and *'mental impairment'*.

The following definitions may be of value:

Learning disabilities

A person with learning disabilities is a person who because of **developmental intellectual handicap**, and regardless of other handicaps, requires extra help to experience an ordinary life, maintain good health, benefit from educational opportunities to maximise skills and minimise deficits.

Severe mental impairment (Mental Health Act 1983)

A state of arrested or incomplete development of the mind which includes severe impairment of intelligence and social functioning, and is associated with abnormally aggressive or seriously irresponsible conduct on the part of the person concerned.

Mental impairment

A state of arrested or incomplete development of mind (not amounting to severe impairment) which includes significant impairment of intelligence and social functioning, and is associated with abnormally aggressive or seriously irresponsible conduct.

The distinction between *'severe mental impairment'* and *'mental impairment'* is one of degree. The assessment of the level of impairment is a matter for clinical judgement.

Thus, under the *Mental Health Act 1983,* compulsory admission to hospital is not appropriate for people with learning disabilities unless there are **associated behavioural problems**, i.e. abnormally aggressive or seriously irresponsible conduct or mental illness.

The *Mental Health Act* also states that mental impairment (as well as psychopathic disorder) must also be amenable to medical — i.e. psychiatric — treatment, so that it is likely to alleviate or prevent a deterioration of the condition.

Children and the Mental Health Act 1983

Finally, one should note that while the Act also applies to children under the age of sixteen, it is rarely applied, for two reasons:

- There are alternatives, such as care proceedings, or for the child to be made a ward of court.

- Parents have powers until the child reaches the age of sixteen, or the age of eighteen if the child is not capable of consent.

These points also apply to children with learning disabilities.

Specific Sections of the Mental Health Act 1983

Community orders

(a) Short-term orders

Sections 135 and 127

Informal admission is available under the *Mental Health Act 1983* with consent, but the individual concerned may not be capable of giving consent. As a result, a situation may arise where there is clear evidence that an adult with learning disabilities is at risk in the community, or is being subjected to physical or emotional abuse, but where social services are powerless to remove that person from the harmful environment unless the person expresses a wish to be removed.

Two provisions of the Act may offer a short-term solution. Under **Section 135** (warrant to search for and remove patients), an approved social worker, who believes that someone is suffering from a mental disorder and is unable to care for himself or herself, or is being ill-treated, can apply to a magistrate for a warrant. This allows a police officer to take the person to a place of safety for up to 72 hours.

Section 127 of the Act makes it a criminal offence to wilfully neglect or ill-treat a person suffering from a mental disorder.

Unfortunately, prosecutions are rarely brought under this Section as evidence can be difficult to obtain; also, it does not offer any long-term solution, as a prosecution does not result in the removal of the victim from the situation which was harmful.

(b) Long-term orders

Section 7

Guardianship is an area where there is much confusion. Many parents believe, in error, that they continue as their child's guardian after the child reaches the age of eighteen.

Once people with learning disabilities reach the age of eighteen, they are, in the eyes of the law, adults.

As adults, they are entitled to make their own decisions about where they should live, how they should spend their money, their personal and sexual relationships, whether they should have medical treatment, and so on.

This may lead to problems, as the person may be unable to understand the issues involved or to make those decisions. Unfortunately the law does not provide an answer to the dilemmas which can arise. In practice, decisions are often sensibly made by carers, professionals and family, but these do not have the force of law.

The *Mental Health Act* offers a limited form of guardianship, i.e. **Section 7**. However, this section applies to very few people with learning disabilities since it only relates to people with one or more of the forms of mental disorder as defined under Section 1 of the *Mental Health Act 1983*.

If someone is eligible for guardianship, the powers of the guardian are limited to three specific areas. The guardian has the right to:

- require the person to live in a specified place

- require the person to attend for medical treatment

- require access to the person by a social worker or doctor.

Note that medical (psychiatric) treatment cannot be forced.

On the whole, Section 7 is infrequently used. (Also see *Mental Health Act 1995* below.)

Mental Health (Patients in the Community) Act 1995

There has been much concern by the public regarding the care of people with mental health problems in the community, who have killed or injured (Ben Silcock and Christopher Clunis are examples of high-profile cases). This has been fuelled by the amount of media coverage. The result of this has to a large extent contributed to the *Mental Health Act 1995*.

Problem areas

The *Mental Health Act 1995* came into force on 1 April 1996. The amendments have not generally been welcomed by any of the professional health bodies.

The Royal College of Psychiatrists was keen to introduce a Community Treatment Order and a Community Supervision Order. The aim was to provide further powers to professionals with respect to patients who stopped taking their medication and were known to relapse. These orders were not implemented.

Another area of concern expressed particularly by approved social workers, was the lack of power to convey (i.e. to use force if necessary) patients on a Section 7 (Guardianship Order):

- to a place of designated treatment

- to their place of designated residence.

This has resulted in an under-use of this order. The new Act now provides for this.

The changes

The *Mental Health Act 1995* has three main elements:

1   **After-care under supervision: Supervised Discharge (Section 25a)**
Essentially to ensure Section 117 After-Care services and to provide formal supervision after discharge.

2   **Absence without leave (Section 18)**
Removes the 28-day limit on returning patients who abscond whilst on a long-term Section. The period is now extended to six months or to the end of the period of detention, whichever is longer. If the Section has lapsed, the patient may be detained for a week for the Responsible Medical Officer to examine for renewal.

3   **Leave of absence from Hospital (Section 17)**
Extends the period during which patients can be on leave to the end of their current Section. In the case of patients who have been detained for a year or more, this could mean that they are granted leave of absence for up to a year.

Care programme approach

All patients who are discharged from hospital (**whether Sectioned or not**) should only be discharged after:

(i)   the **risks** of discharge have been fully assessed

(ii)   a **plan** setting out the after-care provisions (essentially incorporating the elements of Guardianship Order) has been agreed

(iii)   a **key** worker has been allocated

(iv)   there are in place **systematic** arrangements for regular review of the after-care.

The above (i–iv) is known as the **Care Programme Approach**.

Section 117

Section 117 of the *Mental Health Act 1983* places a joint legal duty on health and social services to provide after-care for patients who are discharged from hospital if they have been detained under Sections 3, 37 or 37/41.

The after-care should incorporate all the elements of the Care Programme Approach (see above). However, there is no obligation on a patient to accept the after-care. The patient has a legal right to refuse it.

Supervised discharge (Section 25a)

Since 1 April 1996, a patient's Responsible Medical Officer has been able to make an application to the health authority that is responsible for Section 117 after-care to place a patient on Supervised Discharge.

The main difference now is that **greater power** (to convey) for mental health professionals is provided. However, there are **fewer resources** to implement such powers.

The conditions for supervised discharge are:

(i)   the patient is already detained on Section 3, 37, 48 or 17 (Leave of Absence) but not Section 41

(ii)   the patient is suffering from one of the forms of mental disorder

(iii)   The patient is aged 16 or over

(iv)   there is substantial risk of serious harm to

–   the health or safety of the patient, or

–   the safety of others

(v)   there is risk of serious exploitation

(vi)   that by placing the patient on Supervised Discharge it is likely to help ensure after-care services.

Supervision Register

A patient who presents a substantial risk of harm to themselves or others should be placed on the Supervision Register.

Consent

Definition

For valid consent to exist, there are five essential elements. The competent patient (Cp.), (i.e. 'capable of understanding the nature, the purpose and likely effects of treatment' — *Mental Health Act* definition) who is given information (I) such that the result is the patient understanding the treatment (U). If there is an 'understanding patient' (U) and a voluntary situation between doctor and the patient (V) which results in a 'positive' decision by the patient (D), then valid consent exists. If one element is missing, then valid consent does not exist.

Model for valid consent

$$Cp + I > U$$

$$U + V > D$$

Consent to treatment

Under common law, no treatment can be given to a voluntary patient without his or her valid consent.

The *Mental Health Act 1983* introduced provisions to serve two purposes:

1   to give authority for certain treatments to be given without consent

2   to safeguard psychiatric patients' interests in relation to treatment procedures.

Consent and learning disabilities

Consent is concerned with choosing between two or more options. For people with learning disabilities such choices largely involve issues of lifestyle and social matters, not medical questions.

Children and consent

Children with learning disabilities have the same procedures available to them as children of normal intelligence. The parents make consent decisions by proxy or 'surrogate consent'. If the parents are not available or are incompetent, then procedures of wardship or reception into care are available.

The law dictates that, at the age of sixteen, a child can give informed consent, although he/she is still a minor. Some of those with learning disabilities will not

118

be able to give consent and will be described as legally incompetent. This happens not only to people with learning disabilities, but also to those with long-term and disabling mental illnesses — some following head injury — and those with dementia.

As health care professionals, we support the idea of shared decision-making with adults. With children, there is a shortfall in recognising their rights to autonomy. The *Children Act 1989* failed to make any serious commitment to such rights of autonomy, only limiting itself to stating that children's views should be heard; all too frequently even these limited rights are not upheld.

A recently published report from the Institute of Public Policy Research recommends a Code of Practice and includes: children's rights to receive clear and detailed information; to express views; to grant or withhold consent of any aspect of proposed management — provided that the children are considered to be competent by a doctor, acting in good faith. Parental consent would continue to be valid if it was not against the wishes of the child. The Code of Practice will present a major challenge to health care professionals but, until it is made law, the present trend is unlikely to change. However, a significant change occurred with respect to consent and minors following the ruling in the case of Gillick v. W Norfolk and Wisbech AHA, 1985. The decision now allowed minors to consent to taking the contraceptive pill, provided they were assessed as competent by their doctor. Understandably, many parents remain unhappy about the ruling.

Adults and consent

There is a grey area in the law for the adult (18-plus) who cannot give consent. Parents cannot give consent on their behalf, but it is good practice to have their agreement.

Erroneous thinking can occur with respect to people with learning disabilities and the consent process. This group must not be thought of as homogeneous, as, for example, having one set of competencies.

The problem is that the term *'learning disabilities'* covers a wide range of intellectual disabilities from mild to profound. Some generalisations may provide useful guidelines. Many people with mild learning disabilities can give consent and those with moderate learning disabilities can give consent if the choice is simple. Those with severe learning disabilities cannot give consent.

Where consent cannot be given, the matter may need to go to court. In the special cases of sterilisation, abortion and organ donation, the courts must make a ruling for the individual.

Legal competence can be improved in people with learning disabilities. This population requires encouragement to be more autonomous. Consideration must be given to the opportunities that the individual has had for learning in order to make choices in life, and what consequential results have been experienced. It can be difficult to get away from a paternalistic system. One has to consider the risks involved in allowing the client to make a choice.

Types of consent

Consent may take several forms:

Explicit

This is where informed consent is given to something either verbally or in writing. In order for consent to be valid for an operation, a consent form must be signed by the patient who is competent.

Implicit

In this case, consent is implied by lack of objection. This is particularly relevant for people with learning disabilities where the disability is of a moderate to severe degree. Examples include the giving of medication such as oral contraceptives. Other examples occur every day, such as making decisions for the client in what to wear, when to go to the toilet, and so on. 'Acting in good faith' and showing a 'duty of care' are important ethical guidelines.

Prospective

In this type of consent, lifestyle issues and medical questions are included on forms that relatives or parents are requested to sign when their son or daughter goes into respite or long-term care in some establishments. The signature means, for example, that agreement is given for the person with learning disabilities to go riding or have medical treatment, and so on. Prospective consent, however, is invalid and unacceptable, allowing new care-givers to be both judge and jury.

Spurious

This type of consent is implied from the non-response of the client or the client's parents. An example frequently encountered in medical circles is the 'double negative' letter: 'Your son needs an appointment for the ear, nose and throat department, and unless I hear to the contrary, I will make an appointment.'

Making decisions

People with learning disabilities need to learn to make choices from an early age, and need help to experience the consequences of decisions. Parents, care workers and the medical profession need to understand the legal situation, yet, at the same time, the person with learning disabilities needs to feel included in the decision-making process.

It is very important to value the clients we serve and, where decisions are made on their behalf, those decisions should be made with honesty, respect and humility.

Risk-taking

The overwhelming message from previous sections and chapters should be that people with learning disabilities are people first. Even where mental health issues exist, principles of his or her citizen's rights should take priority over protection principles for the individual. However, where behaviour problems, challenging behaviour or psychiatric illness are present, there are additional considerations regarding the protection of others in the wider environment. Risk-taking decisions must be considered by a systematic procedure which weighs up the relative benefits, costs and safeguards required in potentially risky situations.

Duty of care

Staff working with people with learning disabilities are held in law to have a 'duty of care' towards the users of services. The people who use health and social services are entitled to participate in the activities and opportunities available to ordinary citizens, although they may need extra support to enable this to occur. Staff should take reasonable care in all circumstances, but their 'duty of care' includes allowing and encouraging risk-taking. This should be agreed by their employers (Hughes & Gummer, 1989).

The guiding principle is that a risk should be taken unless there is a good reason not to. There is a need to outline the dimensions of risk for the individual and also to have a mechanism for decision-making. Deciding not to take a risk is a decision, too. The costs to the person with learning disabilities of inaction on behalf of staff may be a severe restriction of quality of life and, in some cases, the action may even amount to a 'neglect' of that individual.

Figure 2

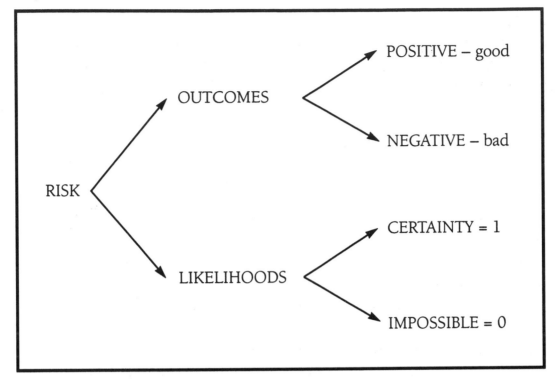

Dimensions of risk

Risk is an occasion when two or more outcomes, whether perceived to be beneficial or harmful, are possible. Something is not a risk if it is certain.

Risk has two variables, as shown in **Figure 2** above: **outcome**, which may be good or bad, and **likelihood**, which may be high or low.

Outcomes have values, degrees of importance or desirability, positive or negative. Ordinarily, outcomes will be expressed in words, although they can be stated in numbers. Numbers will still involve subjective assessments or judgements.

Likelihood can be stated in numbers. It will often be impossible to use exact figures so that assessments of likelihood can be made. The assessment must aim to be an objective estimate of the chances of something happening.

Many risks are taken when working with people with learning disabilities and mental health needs. There are risks involved in the treatment and placement of the person. Will the treatment succeed or fail? Will the person be in danger? Should the person leave the house/hospital/hostel unaccompanied; be encouraged to develop a relationship; learn to drive a car, use the oven, have matches, try horse-riding?

'Many people consider air travel risky, but actually the risk of accident is far greater on the road and should therefore be of more concern. Similarly, the re-offending rate within two years of people released from prison is 50%, whereas of those released from hospital who were convicted of offences, only 25% re-offended'

(Fennell, quoted in Carson, 1991)

although premature release of the mentally ill unjustly causes greater concern amongst the public.

These two examples show that it is better to attempt to evaluate the likely outcomes rather than rely on personal judgement alone.

Remember: we are not always very logical in assessing risks to ourselves and others.

Negative consequences

Consider where hazard might occur:

- distress, annoyance, anger or misunderstanding by members of the public, family, or friends

- distress, annoyance, anger or embarrassment to staff

- distress, annoyance, anger or embarrassment to client

- damage to property

- physical harm to staff, relatives, others or client

- public sanctions – criminal procedures.

Likelihood

It is important not to deny a person a chance, without considering how dangerous it might actually be for that person. It is best to test out the situation in carefully controlled conditions, where possible negative consequences can be minimised. Safeguards should be built in to meet the objective by the least risky means.

Objective

Where there is an element of risk involved in an activity, it must be decided whether the objective is an important addition to the enhancement of independence, freedom and quality of life. The benefits of learning to use public transport could well seem more important to the individual than the possible cost, whereas a decision to take part in bungee-jumping or rock-climbing might be more risky for a person with mental health needs and learning disabilities than the likely benefits would warrant. Or not.

Decision-making

Who decides? Decisions about appropriate goals for a person with learning disabilities should be taken with the person at their individual planning meeting. Where a risk to the client exists, then the group taking the decision needs to be broad: direct-care staff, managers, professionals, advocate and relatives.

If an individual has relatives or an advocate interested in their welfare, it is important to seek their views, but staff should be aware that no-one has a legal right to make a decision on behalf of an adult with learning disabilities.

When a decision to take a risk is made, a plan of implementation and safeguards should be drawn up which will include how progress will be monitored and by whom. Being explicit about costs and benefits to the individual should improve the quality of decision-making and produce judgements that are more ethical.

Dangerousness – a probabilistic approach

It is possible to find predictive risk factors which narrow the probabilities of a particular person being a particular risk (Gunn & Taylor, 1993). Taking an actuarial approach increases the chances of identifying a subgroup of the group causing concern: those voicing threatening or aggressive ideation or verbal abuse to staff or family are more likely to commit offences. This approach reduces the total number of people who are at risk of offending and therefore require more urgent treatment or supervision and tighter communication between services.

Overall, it is only possible to determine probabilities in an individual case. If the priority is to reduce the occurrences of violence, whether in hospital or in the community, then resources have to be put into the 'at risk population' as a whole, since it is not logical to expect professionals to pin-point actual individuals based on predictive factors. Whether a person offends depends on circumstances, support, environment, previous history, course of mental illness, treatability, and generally opportunities to behave in more socially acceptable ways. It is therefore a complex interaction between factors within the individual (which may be more or less knowable by the practitioner), resources available to support the person (in terms of family, friends, services), the reaction of society at large to that person (for example, whether the media are demonising mental illness), and the stigma and provocation the individual might encounter.

Other ethical issues

Citizens' rights

In the USA, there are rights enshrined in law for all citizens, and particular legislation reinforces those rights for people with a disability. Many lawyers, and many in the 'caring' professions, believe that Britain needs a Bill of Rights to protect all citizens — but especially those with disabilities — from discrimination and unfair treatment.

In the absence of 'rights' enshrined in the law of the land, it is possible for services and individuals working in those services to construct their own 'laws' which are often called 'codes of practice'. No group is in as much need of Codes of Practice to safeguard their citizens' rights as people with learning disabilities, who may find it difficult to assert their own rights.

If, in addition, a person with learning disabilities shows signs of mental illness and/or behaviour which challenges those around them, then that person's rights are even more likely to be eroded. The person may suffer from restrictions to their liberty, freedom of movement, and chances to take part in the wider society, and suffer from constraints as to with whom they can have relationships, and how those relationships may be conducted. Such individuals very often have little privacy, few work opportunities, and no control over where they live, how their money is spent or who is making these decisions 'in their best interests'.

This chapter will now address some of the areas where individual rights might be curtailed for people receiving health and social services because of their learning disabilities and mental health needs.

The normalisation philosophy (Wolfensberger, 1972) has led to the de-institutionalisation of services and the stated aim of providing 'an ordinary life'. Because the implementation of this philosophy requires provision of the support necessary for the individual to realise this aim, how far the aim is realised depends on the staff who are employed to carry out that support. The very fact that a person with learning disabilities and mental health needs is in receipt of services puts them in a position where they are dependent on the values and attitudes of those around them. This is the reason why it is so important for staff to spend time examining their own attitudes and for the organisation to formalise a code of ethics to safeguard people's rights.

Sexuality

Historically, the sexuality of people with learning disabilities was dealt with by segregation. Long-stay asylums were built to house people away from society at large and to prevent sexual relationships and reproduction, and men and women were accommodated separately in all-male and all-female wards. The assumptions were that people with learning disabilities were either 'child-like' and therefore lacking in sexual feelings, or 'uncivilised' and therefore unable to control their impulses.

In the last 20 years, the move to 'value' individuals with learning disabilities as members of society has led to a widespread acceptance of their right to an adult sexual identity. The presence of learning disabilities or mental disorder does not of itself preclude emotional maturity; the expression of love, or attraction, and commitment to another person. The United Nations (1971) spelled out people's rights to receive training in social-sexual behaviour, the right to knowledge and the right to express sexual impulses in the same forms that are socially acceptable for others. In the authors' health authority, there is a Sexual Rights Policy (Turk, 1987) which formalises the right of clients to be positively supported by the service to form relationships and express their sexuality.

Having said that, there remains a need to look at how one perceives a person with learning disabilities and mental health needs in terms of their sexuality.

It is often said of people with learning disabilities that they have 'no interest in sex'. This is a statement which must be questioned as it could well stem from a remnant of the 'child-like' model for understanding people with learning disabilities.

On the other hand, it is not uncommon for forms of challenging behaviour to appear sexually motivated because the individual has learnt that sexually inappropriate behaviour produces the response which he or she is seeking.

The staff response could be attention, distress or avoidance of that individual. Again, how one understands the message is crucial and may be based on our own biases. The message can be interpreted as 'illness', challenge, sexual attraction, a need for affection, or a random illogical, unpredictable urge.

How staff feel about people with learning disabilities expressing themselves sexually is very influential in the self-concept of individuals and how they view their own sexuality. Not acknowledging someone's sexual needs may reduce problems for staff, but will be damaging to the individual's personal growth, as well as infringing their rights.

Sexual abuse

While people with learning disabilities have a right to express their sexuality, they have a complementary right to be protected from sexual abuse and exploitation. This right is reinforced by criminal law on rape, assault and consent. All staff should be aware that they have a duty to report an allegation of sexual abuse, and this obligation overrides their duty to keep a confidence. People with learning disabilities and mental health needs are more at risk of sexual abuse than most members of society (Brown & Turk, 1992).

Substitute legal decision-making and representation

There is a well-recognised need for reform in the present law to make up for deficiencies in:

- **public law**: to protect vulnerable people from abuse and neglect

- **private law**: for resolving disputes or uncertainties between individuals about their care, or generally to legitimise and regularise the substitute decision making practice which regularly takes place.

Finance

'Mental disorder' is defined in the *Mental Health Act 1983* as meaning 'mental illness, arrested, incomplete development of mind, psychopathic disorder and any other disorder or disability of mind'. The Court of Protection will supervise a mentally-disordered person's finances when an application is supported by a medical certificate.

Benefits

The *Social Security (Claims and Payments) Regulations 1987* are less stringent. Where claimants are 'unable for the time being to act' for themselves, the DSS will appoint a person to receive benefits on their behalf. The decision as to whether an appointee is necessary is made by the DSS without medical evidence if the claimant is unable to act because 'they do not have the mental ability to understand and control their own affairs'.

Confinement

Confinement means physical methods of keeping a person in one place. Some methods of confinement must not be used without independent authorisation (for example, the Mental Health Act Commission). These methods include restraint by tethering a person to a bed or chair, holding them down, locking them in a room, or using electronic monitoring. Such confinement is not reasonable unless 'it is essential to prevent an immediate risk of serious harm to that person or others.'

Police questioning

Under the *Police and Criminal Evidence Act 1984*, there is a Code of Practice for police to follow for people with learning disabilities. If the police suspect that someone has learning disabilities, they cannot interview that person except in the presence of an 'appropriate adult', who may be a social worker, relative or any responsible adult who is not employed by the police.

Advocacy

Advocacy is about being able to make personal choices. A person with learning disabilities and mental health needs should be given the opportunity to assert their own point of view based on their preferences, wishes and feelings. An independent advocate for a client can help the individual to express his or her personal concerns and aspirations, and find ways to understand, respond and represent that person's interests as if they were their own.

Selecting and training advocates — who enter a one-to-one relationship treated as friendship to support the individual, whilst remaining independent of service provision — is the challenge.

References and further reading

Bingley, W. (1987) The mentally handicapped person as citizen. In: E. Alves (Ed.) *Mental Handicap and the Law*. London: British Psychological Society for the Division of Criminological and Legal Psychology.

Brown, H. & Turk, V. (1992) Defining sexual abuse as it affects adults with learning disabilities. *Mental Handicap,* **20**, (2), 44–48.

Carson, D. (1990) *Risk Taking in Mental Disorder*. Southampton: SLE Publications Ltd.

Carson, D. (1991) *Risk Taking in Health and Social Services*. Southampton: Faculty of Law, University of Southampton.

Craft, A. (Ed.) (1986) *Mental Handicap and Sexuality: Issues and perspectives*. Tunbridge Wells: DJ Costello Publishers.

Edwards, P. & Co. Solicitors. (1995) *A Short Guide to the Mental Health Act (Patients in the Community)*. 5th Edition.

Gunn, J. & Taylor, P. (Eds.) (1993) *Forensic Psychiatry: Clinical, legal and ethical issues*. London: Butterworth-Heinemann.

Gostin, L. (1985) *Mental Health Services and the Law*. London: Shaw.

The Law Commission of Great Britain (1993) *Mentally Incapacitated Adults and Decision Making: A new jurisdiction*. London: HMSO.

Hughes, A. & Gummer, T. (1989) *Risk-taking Policy: Services for people with learning difficulties*. London: Lewisham and North Southwark Health Authority.

Mencap (1989) *Report of the Working Party on the Legal, Medical and Ethical issues of Mental Handicap: Competency and consent to medical treatment*. London: Mencap.

Mental Health Act (1983) London: HMSO.

MIND (National Association for Mental Health) (1993) *Evidence to The Royal Commission on The National Health Service with Regard to Services for Mentally Handicapped People*. London: MIND.

NHS Executive HSG (94), 27 (10.05.94) *Guidelines on the Discharge of Mentally Disordered People and their Continuing Care in the Community*.

Perske, R. (1991) *Unequal Justice*. Nashville: Abingden Press.

Turk, V. (1987) *Sexual Rights: Services for people with a mental handicap*. London: Lewisham and North Southwark Health Authority. Revised by: Hughes, A. & Gummer, T. (1993) *Sexual Rights Policy for Residential Services*. London: Mental Health Unit, Guy's and Lewisham NHS Trust.

United Nations (1971) *Declaration of General and Special Rights of the Mentally Handicapped*. New York: UN Department of Social Affairs.

Whelton, M. & Mann, (1993) *Mental Handicap and the Law*. London: Mencap.

Wolfensberger, W. (1972) *The Principles of Normalisation in Human Services*. Toronto, Canada: National Institute on Mental Retardation.

THE MENTAL HEALTH NEEDS OF CHILDREN WITH LEARNING DISABILITIES

Jeremy Turk

The presence of learning disabilities puts a child at risk of:

● being more dependent on others for help in acquiring basic skills

● being more prone to physical difficulties

● being more prone to emotional and behavioural disturbance

● being more prone to social stigmatisation and its consequences.

In addition the family is put at risk of:

● psychological difficulties in siblings and parents

● marital disharmony.

Young people who have learning disabilities have multiple needs:

● those relating to their learning disabilities

● those relating to their age

● those relating to the impact of their learning disabilities on the family.

Because of this, a multitude of services and professionals is usually involved in an attempt to address the individual's special needs adequately and to promote as normal development as possible. There is also the need for intervention to prevent the development of secondary handicaps to which the individual may be rendered more prone because of their learning disabilities, the cause of their learning disabilities, or their social and educational inadequacies (Turk, 1996a).

Children with learning disabilities can be viewed as children at risk — from biological, psychological and social factors which interact — hence the need for intervention and support in all these areas.

Needs

The needs of a young person with learning disabilities include:

- medical

- emotional

- cognitive

- behavioural

- educational

- social

- familial.

Different services predominate in their contribution at different ages. Throughout preschool years health services undertake a major role, involving paediatricians and Child Development Teams. In some districts, jointly-funded multidisciplinary services provide educational and social input to preschoolers as well. In the school years educational services undertake most support, whether this be within special schools for children with moderate or severe learning difficulties, or by means of extra input within mainstream classrooms, ensured by the undertaking of a 'Full Assessment' leading to a *Statement of Educational Needs* ('statementing'). This legal document should outline the child's educational needs and what special educational support is required to meet them. The document can also list desirable inputs from health and social services. The presence of a Statement ensures educational provision until nineteen years of age — not just the usual sixteen. Thereafter, responsibility for individuals with learning disabilities falls mainly on social services. However, throughout childhood and adolescence there is continuous availability of specialist psychiatric and psychological services for young people, and occasionally highly-specialised teams for young people with learning disabilities who have mental health problems. Also, further education courses ensure availability of learning opportunities well into adulthood.

Multidisciplinary assistance

Essential components of helping a child with learning disabilities comprise:

Medical

- Investigation of possible causes:

    - may have genetic counselling implications for individual and family

    - may highlight likely physical problems requiring intervention (physical phenotype)

    - may provide information on likely developmental and behavioural profiles and thus likely challenges to be faced (behavioural phenotype). (Turk & Sales, 1996)

- Evaluation and treatment of present medical conditions.

- Evaluation and treatment of associated sight or hearing (sensory) problems.

- Assessment for possible psychiatric syndromes found commonly in young people with learning disabilities:

    - autistic spectrum disorders (pervasive developmental disorders) (Lord & Rutter, 1994)

    - hyperkinetic syndrome (attention deficit hyperactivity disorder). (Cameron & Hill, 1996)

- Assessment for and treatment of epilepsy.

Psychological

- Encouragement of optimal development through:
    - comprehensive evaluation of individual profile of cognitive strengths and needs

    - early intervention programmes (such as Portage).

- Evaluation of, and early intervention for, developing challenging behaviours (such as aggression, self-injury) by means of a behavioural functional analysis.

- Counselling/psychotherapy (cognitive, behavioural, psychodynamic) for individual and/or family.

133

Educational

- Thorough evaluation of child's special educational needs.

- Completion of Statement in collaboration with individual, parents, local education authority and other involved professionals.

- Provision of education appropriate to individual's profile of strengths and needs.

- Regular review of appropriateness of provision.

- Availability of specialist services and support for classroom-based behavioural difficulties.

Familial (Turk, 1996b)

- Explanation of nature, chronicity and implications of child's learning disabilities to parents in simple terms.

- Facilitation of familial grieving.

- Continuing availability of support for parents and siblings.

Social

- Welfare benefits.

- Respite care services.

- Holiday and leisure schemes.

- Parent and family support groups (such as MENCAP, 'syndrome societies').

- Contact-a-family.

- Share-a-family.

Long term

- Discussion with individual and family regarding accommodation, occupation and safety.

Prevalence

There is an increased prevalence of emotional and behavioural disturbance in children with learning disabilities compared with their non-learning-disabled peers. This is due to a combination of biological, psychological and social factors. Thus, the following percentages of children have been found (Rutter *et al.*, 1970) to have an identifiable psychiatric disorder:

- 7% of children in the general population

- 12% of children with a physical disorder or disability

- 33% of children with a brain dysfunction

- 50% of children with severe learning disabilities.

Causes of learning disabilities

It is important to distinguish between:

- the cause of the child's long-term disability ('aetiology')

- the cause of the problem (such as challenging behaviour) which has triggered concern.

Causes of learning disabilities are discussed in Chapter X.

Availability of information on aetiology for the individual and family is of critical importance because of:

- the individual and family's basic right to know

- relief from uncertainty regarding the cause of the disabilities

- relief from the guilt that family and/or social factors were the cause of the learning disabilities or developmental or behavioural disturbance

- facilitation of grief resolution

- focusing towards the future

- essential genetic counselling where appropriate for the entire extended family

- instigation of interventions relevant to strengths and needs

- potential for identifying with and belonging to a support group.

Causes of emotional and behavioural problems in young people with learning disabilities

There are many causes of emotional and behavioural problems in young people with learning disabilities. Usually several of these will be responsible for the difficulties faced by any one child.

Constitutional

As with any young person, the individual's temperament, which is itself strongly genetically determined, will contribute substantially towards *how* the child reacts to experiences, and thus the nature and intensity of emotional or behavioural disturbance. Also, the presence of a specific genetic cause (such as Fragile-X syndrome or Prader-Willi syndrome) will determine what developmental and behavioural challenges are likely to be encountered.

Medical

Behavioural disturbance may the consequence of a medical condition; for example, diabetes or epilepsy. It may also be a sign of physical discomfort in a child unable to communicate effectively; for example, in the presence of severe pain due to appendicitis or a fractured bone. Self-injury in the form of hitting the side of the head is a well-recognised presentation of middle ear infection (otitis media). Epilepsy can present as disturbed behaviour even when full consciousness is maintained. Psychiatric disorder will often present with challenging behaviour and, although serious psychiatric conditions such as schizophrenia and manic depression are rare in children with learning disabilities, they are witnessed more often in this group than in children with average intellectual functioning. Brain damage may be a cause of both the learning disabilities and the behavioural disturbance. Medication can be a contributor as well.

Developmental

Behaviour may be appropriate for the developmental stage reached. It is often the discrepancy between the young person's progressing physical size, strength and motor skills, and their limited intellectual and social capacities which creates problems.

Cognitive

It is not 'things' themselves which disturb us but the view we take of them. Thus, the reaction of others to the individual's disabilities is crucial, but so is the reaction of the

136

individual with learning disabilities to their perception of the stigma associated with having disability and their perceptions of other's reactions. This explains why personal counselling and public education must always go hand in hand.

Familial

Emotional or behavioural disturbance in a young person with learning disabilities may be an understandable reaction to family tensions, psychopathology or expressed emotion. This may take the form of a reaction to persisting familial grief or chronic sorrow, or to parental anxieties regarding the past, present or future, or intra-familial conflict or inconsistency.

Social

Problems may be the understandable reaction to life events, persisting communication difficulties and the associated frustration, social deprivation, abuse or neglect, institutionalisation or infantilisation (being treated unnecessarily childishly).

Educational

Educational programmes pitched at either too high or too low a level may contribute to emotional and behavioural disturbance because of either boredom or frustration and upset. The educational placement itself may be contributory. Learning with a disabled peer group may expose children with learning disabilities to inappropriate and maladaptive behaviours. Conversely, learning with a more able group of classmates may highlight just how disabled children are to themselves as well as leaving them open to teasing, bullying and social isolation.

Maladaptive learning

All the above causes can interact with a child's propensity to learn inappropriate and maladaptive responses to situations where there is a problem in gaining attention, avoiding social interaction or difficult tasks, or in getting his or her own way.

Multidisciplinary interventions for problems encountered

Medical

Epilepsy can further aggravate learning disabilities and can cause, or exacerbate behavioural problems. Its presence in association with severe learning disabilities is a potent vulnerability factor predisposing towards psychological problems. Anticonvulsant medication should be combined with psychological approaches.

Physical disfigurement as part of a physical phenotype may cause profound distress in the child and family requiring long-term psychological support.

Psychiatric disturbance may occasionally warrant medical intervention, such as the confirmed benefits of stimulant medication, such as methylphenidate (Ritalin) for hyperkinetic disorder (Payton *et al.*, 1989).

Psychological

The impact on family functioning of the presence of a child with learning disabilities may be profound. This in turn may aggravate the child's problems. Thus, family therapy may be indicated. More often, behavioural approaches will be appropriate, although other family members will need to be included to act as co-therapists. Behavioural approaches are not without limitations, which must be born in mind while devising and undertaking such interventions. Commonly experienced problems include:

- high response specificity to environment in which programme is undertaken, i.e. the improvement may not manifest in different settings or with different individuals

- difficulties in generalising improvements to other settings

- need for long-term intensive continuation of behavioural programmes to maintain benefits and prevent relapse.

Educational

Special education, whether in special school or with specialist input within a mainstream school, is of primary importance in addressing the needs of the learning-disabled child. Teaching programmes must be tailored to the child's developmental level and must be mindful of associated difficulties such as autism. This would require a particular emphasis on structured and predictable programmes, with a focus on the multiple qualitative impairments in social functioning, language, and

138

ritualistic tendencies which are the hallmarks of the condition. Certain causes of learning disabilities may create specific requirements for classroom adaptations; for example, the gaze aversion, sequential information-processing difficulties and numeracy problems often witnessed in Fragile-X syndrome.

Attention deficits

Attention deficits and overactivity are common in children with learning disabilities and are often consistent with the individual's developmental level. Sometimes they may be particularly marked. There is evidence that certain genetic causes of learning disabilities are more likely to lead to these difficulties; for example, Fragile-X syndrome, Smith-Magenis syndrome and Sanfillipo syndrome. The following features require careful consideration:

- **Inattentiveness**
  Is the child unable to concentrate for any length of time, even on enjoyed activities?

- **Restlessness**
  Is the child unable to stay seated for any length of time? Is he or she always up-and-down from his/her seat even during mealtimes and other enjoyed activities?

- **Fidgeting**
  Is the child constantly twiddling his/her fingers and toes and shuffling around on his/her bottom when seated?

- **Overactivity**
  Is he/she always on the go?

- **Impulsiveness**
  Is he/she the sort of child who always acts first and thinks later — if at all? Is he/she unable to wait before doing something?

- **Distractibility**
  Even when he/she does concentrate, is this extremely fragile so that even the slightest distraction breaks concentration?

If all these features are present in a wide range of settings, irrespective of whom the child is with and what time it is ('all-pervasiveness') then the child may have hyperkinetic disorder (or attention deficit hyperactivity disorder). This condition is known to have a biological basis related to delays in maturation of certain parts of the brain. As well as requiring specialist educational and psychological input, individuals often benefit from judicious use of stimulant medications such as methylphenidate, but these must always be prescribed and monitored by a professional experienced in this highly-specialised field, who has undertaken a thorough and appropriate evaluation. Contrary to earlier beliefs, there is now evidence that some children with even severe learning disabilities can respond beneficially to concentration-enhancing approaches, including stimulant medication.

Adolescence

Separation and individuation issues are particularly complex for adolescents with learning disabilities. The ongoing struggle between autonomy and dependency coexists with practical issues such as the development of sexual awareness and drives, and the need to ensure that individuals are protected from abuse and exploitation. Inability to achieve true independence from the family may be a cause of depression and anger.

Summary

Young people with learning disabilities usually have multiple special needs which include an increased likelihood of emotional and behavioural disturbance. Biological, psychological and social factors all interact and all require careful assessment and intervention in order to maximise the child's welfare and to minimise the risks of avoidable secondary handicaps. Inadequate knowledge, resources and support (practical and emotional) renders young people with learning disabilities at risk of further distress and disadvantage. Hence, close collaborative work by multiple agencies with the family throughout and beyond childhood is necessary to ensure optimal outcome.

References and further reading

Cameron, M. & Hill, P. (1996) Hyperkinetic disorder: Assessment and treatment. *Advances in Psychiatric Treatment, 2*, 94–102.

Lord, C. & Rutter, M. (1994) Autism and pervasive developmental disorders. In: M. Rutter, E. Taylor & L. Hersov (Eds.), *Child and Adolescent Psychiatry: Modern Approaches*. Oxford: Blackwell Scientific.

Payton, J. B., Burkhart, J. E., Hersen, M. & Helsel, W. J. (1989) Treatment of ADDH in mentally retarded children: A preliminary study. *Journal of the American Academy of Child and Adolescent Psychiatry, 28*, 761–767.

Rutter, M., Graham, P. & Yule, W. (1970) A neuropsychiatric study in childhood. *Clinics in Developmental Medicine,* No. 35/36. London: Heinemann/Spastics International Medical Publications.

Turk, J. (1996a) Tertiary prevention of childhood mental health problems. In: T. Kendrick, A. Tylee & P. Feeling (Eds.) *The Prevention of Mental Illness in Primary Care.* Cambridge: Cambridge University Press. 265–280.

Turk, J. (1996b) Working with parents of children who have severe learning disabilities. *Clinical Child Psychology & Psychiatry,* **1**, 583–598.

Turk, J. & Sales, J. (1996) Behavioural phenotypes and their relevance to child mental health professionals. *Child Psychology & Psychiatry Review,* **1**, 4–11.

DISENTANGLING THE NATURE OF AUTISM

Jill Bradshaw, Ella Brent and Susan Macdonald

This chapter will look at defining autism and the implications for supporting individuals who fall within the **autistic spectrum of disorders.**

To enable provision of the right support for an individual with autism, carers need to know and understand the underlying impairments associated with autism, how these individuals experience their environments, and how these impact on their behaviour.

Developing an understanding of autism

Autism is a perplexing disorder and our understanding of it has evolved greatly over recent decades, though many questions remain unanswered. We now know much more about the underpinning impairments of autism but continue to search for the exact sites of the brain where the impairments lie and how they operate.

Media attention through films like *Rain Man* and television documentaries have brought autism and its issues to a wider audience. This, however, has not de-mystified the complexity of the disorder, nor has it dispelled all the myths surrounding autism amongst the general public.

Many continue to view those with autism as having special gifts/talents, a dislike of touch from others and being prone to temper tantrums. Though these points may be true of some people with autism, they omit the vital understanding of the underlying communication and social impairments of autism.

A historical picture of autism

The word autistic appeared in the 1940s and was used by two independent pioneers, Leo Kanner (USA) and Hans Asperger (Vienna) working with children. Autistic comes from the Greek word 'autos' meaning 'self' and both men used the word to encapsulate the children's inability to relate to others. The children appeared to ignore and disregard what was going on around them. Instead, they related to objects and could occupy themselves for hours playing with items in a repetitive manner. They were rigid in their interests and showed a marked 'desire for sameness'. Some had isolated talents which were quite extraordinary.

For many years the predominant theories which explained these children's autistic behaviours were held by the psychoanalysts. The term 'childhood schizophrenia' was used to label a large range of childhood psychiatric disorders and there was much debate and disagreement on autism. It was one of these psychoanalysts, Bruno Bettleheim, who in the 1960s saw the underlying cause of autism to be the 'frozen' parents' inability to emotionally bond and interact with their child (particularly the mother).

Today it is accepted that autism is not a result of emotional deprivation and thankfully, parents are no longer blamed. Scientists in many fields continue to look for the causes of autism. Advances in the understanding of the brain's pathology may lead us one day to an area where autism can be 'located' or seen to operate within the brain. Research does indicate that there is likely to be no one single cause of autism, but it may operate in combination with genetic or other factors.

What is autism?

Autism is seen as a continuum or spectrum of disorders. People with autism fall along a continuum of diverse characteristics, all resulting from the underlying triad of impairments:

- impairment in verbal and non-verbal communication

- impairment in two-way social interaction (relationships)

- impairment of imaginative skills and limited interests.

The diagnosis of autism is made through recognising patterns of behaviour from early life. Both the *Diagnostic and Statistical Manual* (DSM-III-R) of the American Psychiatric Association and the *International Classification of Diseases* (ICD 10) issued by the World Health Organisation, use the Triad of Impairments, as a basis for diagnosis.

The signs of autism are difficult to detect in infancy and may go unnoticed by parents, though they often report that looking back, they knew something was wrong. As the child gets older, the developmental milestones may be late or, in some cases, absent (i.e. no speech is developed) and often then parents begin to question the child's catalogue of odd behaviours and strange lack of interest in others.

Asperger's syndrome

Asperger's original patients had been more able than those of Kanner and today Asperger's syndrome refers to those individuals with autism who have normal or above normal intelligence.

People with Asperger's syndrome have impairments in reciprocal social interactions resulting in a solitary lifestyle, language problems and difficulties with non-verbal communication.

Their all-absorbing narrow interests make them stand out, and their lack of sensitivity to others' capacity for discussing these favourite subjects make most encounters one-sided and tedious.

Their difficulty in understanding that others have different thoughts and feelings from their own makes the imposition of their routines and interests on others automatic.

The prevalence of autism

Autism occurs across all cultures and all social classes, dispelling the theories of the 1960s which saw autism as a middle-class problem. Autism affects approximately three times more boys than girls (Wing & Gould, 1979).

The prevalence of autism using the narrow classical autistic criteria gives rates of two to four children in every 10,000 (Gilberg *et al.*, 1986).

Wing and Gould (1979), using a wider definition of the autistic spectrum, found the prevalence of the triad of impairments to be 22 in every 10,000 children. Similar findings elsewhere, using the same wider definition of the autistic spectrum, have shown the prevalence to be 15–20 in every 10,000 children.

Since autism is a rare disorder, you would not expect to see more than one child in a family with autism, but this is not the case. Autism appears to 'run in the family', with two per cent of siblings of autistic children being diagnosed as autistic. This may highlight the link between autism and inherited genes.

Approximately one-third of people with autism have moderate to severe learning disabilities. A further third have mild learning disabilities, and the remainder have normal or above normal intelligence (Asperger's syndrome).

Autism is increasingly likely to occur in those who have severe learning disabilities, though the causes for the association between autism and learning disabilities is not clear.

The causes of autism

Autism is not an illness, nor is it curable. The exact causes of autism are not clear, though biological/genetic research into autism is providing more clues as to its origin.

No one medical condition can be seen to be the cause of autism, though a number of links have been made with the following conditions:

- Fragile-X syndrome

- Rett's syndrome

- phenylketonuria

- tuberous sclerosis

- viral infections (such as congenital rubella)

- difficulties experienced during pregnancy/birth

- mother over 35 years.

Though these prenatal and postnatal causes are only evident in a minority of children with autism, they may well be signs of the abnormality and not the cause of it.

There appears to be no single cause of autism, rather a combination of genetic and biological factors.

The triad of impairments

This section aims to explore in greater detail the difficulties people with autism experience in each of the three areas within the triad. No two people will present with exactly the same strengths and needs within each of these areas. Individuals may also have more difficulties within one of the triad of impairments than in another. All people with autism will have some difficulties in each area. People do develop skills and may learn strategies to reduce the effects of their difficulties.

Impairment in verbal and non-verbal communication

There is a range of skills in communication. In terms of expression, there are some people who do not communicate using speech or gestures but who indicate their needs by going to get what it is they desire; for example, going to the kitchen if they are hungry. Some may be completely reliant on other people to interpret their needs. Some people with autism communicate by using single words, whilst others use short phrases or complete sentences. This may be to indicate needs or include a wider range of communication functions; for example, to request information. Some 60% of people with autism develop speech and of these people, 75% will echo speech (Baltaxe and Simmons, 1981).

Communication development

Frequently, hearing loss is the first thing which is investigated. Autistic children may not focus on speech and therefore the sound of the refrigerator may be of more interest/importance to them than the sounds of people. Children without autism have an inherent interest in speech over non-speech sounds (Klin, 1991).

Joint attention difficulties are often present (Mundy *et al.*, 1990) and children's attention may be difficult to direct. One of the ways in which language develops is by the carer and child looking at the same item and the carer making comments about the item. It also involves the notion of 'interest sharing': that there is a pleasure in this activity. Children with autism often find other people confusing and may not find the experience of 'focusing attention' interesting, particularly when there are other distractions. If attention is difficult to direct, language learning is at least delayed and sometimes results in children learning incorrect labels for objects; for example, by not looking at the object which the person was talking about.

Pointing is often difficult, as is understanding gestures. Children may not be able to look in the direction of the point and may be looking at the end of the person's finger. They may not use gestures in the same way as other children; for example, not holding out their arms to indicate they wish to be picked up. Children may lead other people to what they want rather than pointing. They may also direct the person's hand to what they want by holding the person's hand and placing it on the object (Frith, 1989).

Autistic children may develop these skills, but at a later stage than other children. The delay will influence the child's learning of language and difficulties with communication are likely to persist.

Understanding and people with autism

Understanding of words

People with autism often have difficulties in attending to one stimulus out of a number, for example, speech, and may find it very difficult when there are other distractions in the environment. We all find it difficult to listen in very noisy and chaotic environments but people with autism may be particularly affected by internal distractions; for example, the need to arrange items in a particular order. Trying to understand what is being said when the kettle is not in its 'correct' place may be extremely difficult.

People with autism may learn phrases without being able to recognise and separate the constituent words of the phrase into their meanings. Language may have been learnt as a chunk of sounds. Changing the word order may make the sentence meaningless.

Gestures and facial expressions may be difficult for people with autism. Understanding is reliant on the person's knowledge of the intent behind the gesture or expression. If you are not aware of the emotion behind the expression, for example, crying, it may just seem to be a strange sound. People may have difficulties in recognising that someone is bored from their expression. Difficulties with understanding emotion-related words are frequently noted. This is partly to do with the difficulties in understanding abstract concepts, but also to do with the difficulties people with autism have with understanding and recognising that other people may have thoughts, feelings and beliefs that are different from theirs. This is to do with the concept of 'theory of mind'. Tests have shown that when people with autism are asked to give information about what another person thinks or feels, they frequently give information that is consistent with what they would think given their knowledge and experience, and do not separate this from what others know and experience (Baron-Cohen *et al.*, 1985).

Expression

Difficulties with understanding will be reflected in the person's expressive skills. It is usually the case that people understand more than they are able to express, but this

148

is not necessarily the case in people with autism as they may echo speech. People who use signs may also echo signing. People with autism may use complex sentences but actually only understand some of the words they are using. Facial expressions may not reflect what the person is saying; for example, saying, 'go away' but smiling.

People with autism may not find the process of communication inherently rewarding. They may have repeated experiences of unsuccessful attempts to communicate and be confused about many aspects of the process. This may contribute to people only communicating to make their needs known; for example, to request a drink, but not for the social pleasure that many of us find in engaging in conversation. This will also be reflected in the difficulties people have in learning language and their (frequently) limited vocabularies.

Echoed speech

Echoing may take a number of forms and have a variety of communication functions. Echoing can occur in the following combinations:

- **immediate-exact** – repeating the same phrase just after another has spoken it

- **immediate-modified** – repeating just after another has spoken, but changing the phrase in some way. This could be by repeating only part of the phrase, or by missing out part of the sentence or tense markers

- **delayed-exact** – this is an exact repetition which occurs at a later time; this may be a few seconds later or a few minutes or longer

- **delayed-modified** – the echoed phrase has been changed in some way and is repeated sometime after it has been heard
  (Frith, 1989).

Echoing is a normal process in the learning of language. People with autism often continue to echo speech and have great difficulties in using new sentences which are not echoed. Language may be learnt as chunks without an understanding of how to break language down into its parts or how to use these creatively and flexibly.

Echoing is a skill and it requires an ability to attend selectively to speech and to the speech of one person. It requires the ability to remember and process the sequences of sounds heard and to be able to reproduce these sounds in the same order. This can be done without processing the meaning of the words echoed.

Echoing may have a variety of functions or it may be used without any apparent communicative intent. People may repeat a phrase as a way of taking part in a conversation. It may be used as a request; for example, when asked, 'Do you want a coffee?' the person responds, 'want coffee'. People usually echo more when they are in stressful situations. Echoing also increases when people do not understand what others are saying. Sometimes familiar words are more likely to be repeated.

Phrases are sometimes learnt in association with a particular event. This may or may not be with understanding of what the phrase means. Being in the same or similar situations to those in which the phrase was first learnt may trigger an echo of that phrase.

Recurrent themes can often be observed in an individual's communication. These may be around particular interests or be around people's anxieties. They may be phrases that people use in situations where they are confused about what is happening. People may become 'stuck' in repetitive themes and they can persist in these conversations for a long time once started. Strategies to enable people to switch from repetitive themes must be developed.

An understanding of how the individual communicates is essential in the planning of effective support for people with autism. Individuals should be supported to use their existing skills and to develop functional communication skills. Speech and language therapists will be able to provide assessment information, plan interventions and support staff to implement these changes to the communication environment.

Social impairments

The impairment of reciprocal social interaction refers to the inability to engage in two-way interactions with others and, on a more global level, difficulties forming relationships with others.

Wing and Gould (1979) attempted to measure the degree of social impairment in a group of autistic children and identified three distinctive groups:

- the aloof

- the passive

- the active but odd.

People in the **aloof** group appear withdrawn and do not respond to the situations and speech going on around them. They appear to be in a world of their own. They will only seek out others in order to have simple needs met, and this involves leading the carer to the desired object. Eye contact with others appears to be avoided, as well as physical contact with others, though rough/tumble play or listening to music while being cuddled may be acceptable to some.

150

People in the **passive** group accept social approaches with indifference and will often comply with all requests and therefore could easily be 'led astray'. They have good speech and will answer questions without hesitation and with complete honesty. Social contact is accepted by them as part of life, but is not something which is pursued for pleasure. Difficulties dealing with stresses and changes in routines can cause great anxiety and will result in emotional displays and/or temper tantrums.

People in the **active but odd** group enjoy being with people and touching people. There is no distinction between familiar people and total strangers, and individuals lack the understanding of when a contact with someone is wanted or unwanted, socially appropriate or socially unacceptable, causing great difficulties. This group will be known for their pestering of people and as a result carers will often not let the individual out on their own. People in this group can often show or have a tendency for physical aggression.

People with autism also have difficulties in understanding how other people feel, (imagining), or knowing that other people have different thoughts, beliefs, or interests.

Difficulties using language to communicate

Communication difficulties are also reflected in people's difficulties in understanding the social rules of interactions. However skilled people with autism are in communicating, all people with autism will have some difficulties in using language to communicate.

Impairment of imaginative skills and limited interests

The third of the triad highlights the difficulties people with autism face in terms of developing creative and imaginative skills and having a narrow area of thoughts and behaviours.

As with the other aspects of the triad, it affects people with autism in different ways and to different degrees; for example, as a repetitious conversational topic (always wanting to talk about bus routes) or as repeated behaviours (spinning a coin or rocking).

Autism is thought to affect the way in which people's brains receive and use information affecting all of the five senses.

Faced with huge amounts of information which stimulates each of our senses, we can filter what is useful and what is not. If this mechanism does not work, a person

151

will quickly become overwhelmed with all the competing information. The incoming information will be jumbled, unclear and confused.

Able people seem to have an inbuilt rule to give most attention to things that have some meaning or relevance. When we filter new information we can fit it into what we already know so that it makes sense, even if it is not exactly the same as what we have experienced before. These two methods of 'sorting' new information and updating old information together allows us to **learn flexibly**. People with autism seem to treat and store all information as isolated fragments and are unable to learn flexibly.

This underlying problem explains many difficulties people with autism have in learning and using skills across environments.

If the environment is overwhelming, unpredictable, or under-stimulating, people with autism may cope by engaging in rigid routines and behaviours to reduce the unpredictability and anxiety they experience. These rigid routines and behaviours may be challenging to those caring for individuals with autism.

Support for people with autism

There have been many approaches to the treatment and support of people with autism. New ones are always appearing on the scene while others drift away into obscurity. Approaches to autism arise from the prevailing theories of the nature of autism. With our greater understanding of the underlying triad of impairments, we can be certain that by addressing these, we can enable people with autism to participate more fully in our 'non-autistic world'.

When we cannot communicate or interact with others in a meaningful way, we feel and behave differently. There are also differences in our behaviour between when we understand what is happening and when we do not. There are many parallels between our responses and those of people with autism in these types of situations.

The alternative methods of support advocated here stem from the acknowledgement of the three main areas of difficulty experienced by people with autism: **verbal and non-verbal communication**, **social interaction**, and **restricted activities and interests**.

It is likely that a person who has no idea of what is happening will see any demand from others as unpredictable and intrusive. A person with autism may have to resort to focusing on the only aspects of predictability that there are: meal times, staff/shift changes, and their own repetitive routines/behaviours. The day will probably seem

152

long and stressful for the person with autism, who has no clear idea or understanding of what will happen next. A predictable, structured approach is crucial when supporting people with autism.

Just as we do not like our habits prevented, it is important to remember that these things are very important to people with autism and will require negotiation with them. If these routines/rituals are limiting or harming for a person's development of skills and their quality of life, then ways will need to be developed to find rewarding and appropriate alternative behaviours. The long-term aim should be to reduce these habits and not to eliminate them, but to allow people with autism times and places for these habits (set limits for the person) and ensure that the person with autism understands this (i.e. when they can do it).

There are clear ways we can make strange and unpredictable situations more predictable and as a result less stressful for people with autism. These 'supports' are practical (e.g. visual timetables) and can be developed to make life easier for people with autism, allowing them to know and make choices around their daily lives. Information needs to be present in the environment to inform and remind people of what they will be doing, when, and who will support them in the activity. This can be done in a variety of ways to meet the communication needs of the individual.

When people are this easily distracted, information from language, which is very temporary, can be lost as soon as the person stops speaking. Language is often difficult for people to use, even if it can be understood.

In order to reduce the stress of so many distractions, when supporting people with autism it is important to reduce anything which is irrelevant. The use of very clear language aided by object/visual cues where appropriate will prove very effective in increasing the individual's understanding. When carrying out tasks, often it can be useful to follow universal rules such as starting on the left and finishing on the right. Open-ended creative activities are more difficult than clear tasks with predictable starts and finishes.

By understanding what people with autism are likely to find difficult, we can ensure that we provide helpful environments and support which will maximise their potential.

Conclusion

By addressing the underlying triad of impairments, we can enable people with autism to participate more fully in our 'non-autistic world'.

Communication is a key factor in people's daily lives. It is vital to recognise an individual's communication strengths and needs, the need for predictability and structure and the difficulties with social interactions. Support should be provided on an individual basis, with environments tailored to meet people's needs. This is necessary to enable individuals to learn and use skills and participate in daily living.

References and further reading

American Psychiatric Association: *Diagnostic and Statistical Manual.* DSM III-R, 1987; DSM IV, 1994.

Baltaxe, C. & Simmons, J. (1981) Disorders of language in childhood psychosis. In: J. Darby (Ed.) *Speech Evaluation Psychiatry.* New York: Grine and Statton, 285–329.

Baron-Cohen, S., Leslie, A. M. & Firth, U. (1985) Does the child have a theory of mind? *Cognition,* **21**, 37–46.

Frith, U. (1989) *Autism, Explaining the Enigma.* Oxford: Basil Blackwell.

Gilberg, C. Persson, E. Grufman, M. & Themner, U. (1986) Psychiatric disorders in mildly and severely mentally retarded urban children and adolescents: Epidemiological aspects. *British Journal of Psychiatry,* **149**, 68–74.

Klin, A. (1991) Young autistic children's listening preferences in regard to speech: A possible characterisation of the symptom of social withdrawal. *JADD,* **20** (1).

Mundy, P., Sigman, M., & Kasari, C. (1990) A longitudinal study of joint attention and language development in autistic children. *JADD,* **20** (1).

Williams, D. (1993) *Nobody Nowhere.* Corgi Books.

Williams, D. (1994) *Somebody Somewhere.* Doubleday.

Wing, L. & Gould, J. (1979) Severe impairments of social interaction and associated abnormalities in children: Epidemiology and classification, *JADD,* **9**, 11–30.

Wing, L. (1996) *The Autistic Spectrum: A guide for parents and professionals.* Constable.

World Health Organisation (1993) *The ICD-10 Classification of Mental and Behavioural Disorders: Diagnostic Criteria for Research.* Geneva: WHO.

Video

A is for Autism. Directed by Tim Webb. A Finetake Production for Channel 4, 1992. Available for purchase from the BFI (British Film Institute, Head Office, 21 Stephen Street, London W1 2LN).

This is a short 11-minute animated documentary film about the experience of autism, from the autistic individual's perspective and offers great insight into their condition.

MENTAL HEALTH AND AGEING

Steve Moss

Ageing and learning disabilities

The age structure of the population in most industrialised countries is changing. People are living longer and having fewer children, with the result that the proportion of older people has been steadily rising. This 'greying' of society is predicted to continue well into the twenty-first century, with a consequent pressure on services to older people that is becoming of increasing concern to policy planners. The 'baby boom' shortly after World War II and into the mid-1960s created a population surge which will result in a 'senior boom' which will peak in numbers by the year 2035.

The increasing proportion of elderly people is due not only to changes in birth rate, but to an improvement in life expectancy. One of the main reasons for this has been improvements in the quality of medical care. People are now much more likely to survive serious illness in old age than they were 50 years ago. For people with learning disabilities, many of whom tend to be more susceptible to illness than their non-disabled peers, these medical advances have had an even greater impact. Advances in perinatal care have resulted in a much greater proportion of learning-disabled children surviving the first year of life. Nowadays, the death rate among children with Down syndrome in the first year of life is lower than 10%, compared with 50% earlier in the century. Mortality rates amongst adults has shown similar decline as major causes of death have been brought under control — such as tuberculosis, pneumonia and influenza.

When research on the ageing of this population started to gain momentum in the mid-1970s, the literature abounded with assertions that this was a population with 'special needs', given what was described as the 'double jeopardy' of being both elderly and 'mentally retarded' (Sweeney & Wilson, 1979). Since that time, a number of studies have demonstrated that a population over 50 years of age, with an at least moderate level of disability, does indeed show special characteristics, but that these characteristics do not give the picture one might expect. Rather than being a population with failing health and increasing support needs, most individuals are in basically good health and with good functional skills (Holland & Moss, 1996). The reason for this is that **differential mortality**, i.e. the tendency for the frailer members of a population to die earlier, operates very strongly in this population, and increasingly strongly the more severe the level of disability. Thus, Moss (1991) found, using a major UK learning disabilities register, a constantly-reducing proportion with severe epilepsy over the lifespan; the presence of epilepsy being an indicator of neurological impairment which is associated with early mortality. The reduction over the adult lifespan was caused by the differential mortality of these at-risk individuals, most of whom were severely or profoundly disabled.

For many older people with learning disabilities, the presentation, diagnosis and management of psychiatric disorders in later life will be very similar to the general elderly population. However, this population may present with mental health problems in unusual ways for a variety of reasons including: the effects of the pre-existing learning disabilities and impaired language development; the direct effect of brain dysfunction, due to the presence since conception or early childhood of a severe abnormality of brain development; the increased rates of physical disabilities, sensory impairments and epilepsy which might further complicate the clinical picture; and a lifetime history of living in institutional or unsophisticated living environments. People with learning disabilities may be unable to describe the symptoms they are experiencing, or to appreciate that their abilities or mood have changed. Loss of skills, as occurs in dementia, goes unnoticed or is presumed to be related to the presence of a learning disability (Holland & Moss, 1996). For a practical discussion of issues relating to mental health see Moss et al. (1997).

Psychiatric disorders in the general elderly population

Although there are a number of specific issues relating to older people with learning disabilities, it is important to bear in mind that ageing is a process common to us all. Studies of the general population of elderly people living in the community indicate that this group suffers from definite psychiatric symptoms in a high proportion, perhaps 20% of the over 65s. Their psychiatric symptoms are often accompanied by physical illnesses, and they are often disabled by their symptoms. Some 50% of US hospital and nursing-home beds for the elderly are occupied by psychiatrically-ill elderly people (Gianturko & Busse, 1978), yet the use of psychiatric out-patient services by the elderly is low, and less than five per cent of this age group reside in institutions. It therefore appears that there may be many older people in the community who need psychiatric help but do not receive it.

Two principal reasons have been suggested for this discrepancy between service need and take-up in the community elderly. First, systems of health care have generally evolved on a model more suitable for a younger, more assertive, vigorous and affluent age group, whose disorders tend to be more consistent with traditional organisation of professional and specialist services. Second, complaints of elderly people often do not fit neatly into the compartments (such as 'psychiatric', 'medical' or 'social') which are generally built into a health care system. In elderly people particularly, medical illnesses can mimic psychiatric disorders, which in turn can present as physical problems. Thus, it is frequently found that somatic, rather than psychiatric, symptoms dominate the picture, so that the elderly depressed person may complain only of a headache, backache or joint pains.

Regarding overall prevalence, a minimum level of two per cent is suggested by the fact that data on patient care episodes show at least one-and-a-half per cent of over-65s were under psychiatric care from either in-patient or out-patient services (Hogg, Moss & Cooke, 1988). Much higher estimates come from community surveys of psychiatric morbidity on general practice lists or random samples of the general population. Thus Shepherd *et al.* (1966) found psychiatric morbidity rates within a general practice to be 11% for men and 15% for women.

Depression

This is by far the most common mental health problem in older people. Data varies from study to study, depending on population and criteria, although it is generally thought that 15–20% of elderly people suffer from depressive symptoms (Shamoian, 1985). However, only 15–20% of this depressed group will receive treatment. Shamoian points out that elderly people often deny their depression and are reluctant to seek psychiatric assistance. Their denial and unwillingness to seek assistance is complicated by frequent misinterpretation of the signs and symptoms of depression as disparate symptoms of normal ageing. Severely depressed elderly people show an increased use of medical services; they take more psychotropic medications and are given multiple drugs more often. They see their doctor repeatedly, receive more special investigations, and are admitted to hospital more frequently.

In one major study (Gianturko and Busse, 1978), it was notable that the majority of respondents were able to trace most depressive episodes to specific life events. This finding suggests one should be cautious in generalising results to a population of people with learning disabilities, since for many of these people the course of life events will have been very different from those of the general population.

Dementia

The most obviously age-related mental health problem is dementia. There are a number of different types, of which Alzheimer-type dementia is the most frequent. Alzheimer's disease is associated with a number of characteristic cellular changes which are widely distributed throughout the brain. Apart from Alzheimer's, the other most commonly occurring type is multi-infarct dementia, in which the brain is damaged in a number of localised sites by damaged blood vessels.

The dementia syndrome involves deterioration in many aspects of mental functioning. However, the changes can be summarised under three headings:

- memory

- other cognitive functioning

- emotional changes.

A full diagnosis of dementia under the criteria laid down by the World Health Organisation needs clinical evidence in all three of these areas.

Memory loss involves both short- and long-term memory, although long-term memories are retained longer than the capacity to learn and remember new information. It must be stressed that many older people have poorer memories, but this is usually a benign consequence of ageing, rather than indicative of dementing disease.

Other cognitive functioning refers to a variety of skill areas including the cerebral control of reading, speaking, object recognition and abstract thinking.

Emotional changes observed in dementia may involve wandering/pacing, aggressive behaviour, apathy/loss of drive, depressive symptoms, delusions and hallucinations.

It must be stressed that the diagnosis of Alzheimer's disease, or any other dementia for that matter, involves the ruling out of any other possible cause for the symptoms, as well as an understanding of the significance of the pattern of symptoms. This requires a high level of clinical expertise. Due to the seriousness and poor prognosis of many types of dementia, it is essential that the diagnosis be made only when all the clinical evidence has been properly evaluated.

Alzheimer-type dementia usually begins with mild memory and language disturbances. This stage is followed by more serious symptoms including severe memory loss, disturbances in perception, problems with speech and language and general disorientation. As the disease progresses, functional skills will be lost and the person will become increasingly disorientated. Control over movement will also

160

decline. The person's mental state may also change with depression, delusions, aggression and irritability evident. Towards the end of life, all functional skills will be lost and the person will require total care. Death may result from a number of acute causes, including pneumonia and heart failure.

Two points of great importance must be made with respect to diagnosis:

1   The progressive deterioration must be monitored against the individual's level of functioning before they became ill. Use of population average functioning is not sufficiently accurate, even in the case of the general population. For people with learning disabilities this is clearly crucial, and is one of the reasons why diagnosis in this population can be so problematical — retrospective information on functional level is usually not very reliable unless routine monitoring using a standardised schedule has been carried out over a period of time.

2   A general decline in functioning cannot in itself be taken as an indication of dementia. It is the characteristic pattern of changes which identifies the disorder. Once again, it is stressed that clinical expertise is necessary to identify and diagnose dementia.

Psychiatric problems in older people with learning disabilities

A number of studies have reported important clinical findings relating to the ageing process (see Day & Jancar, 1994, for a review). Affective psychoses (mostly bipolar) tend to start in the over-40s and are more common in women. Paranoid psychoses are more likely to start over the age of 50, sometimes being associated with temporal lobe epilepsy, severe visual and hearing defects and interpersonal difficulties. Day and Jancar (1994) also draw attention to the importance of environmental and social factors in the genesis of mental illness. These include separation from, or death of a parent, loneliness and sudden relocation. These life events can lead to depression and anxiety which can sometimes be mistakenly attributed to dementia.

A study carried out in Oldham looked at a population over age 50 years and with a learning disability. Results found 12 individuals out of a total sample of 105 to have a diagnosable psychiatric condition (apart from dementia), giving an overall prevalence rate of 11·4% (Patel *et al.*, 1993). Most of the disorders detected in this older population were not 'high profile' — neither psychotic, nor within the range of conditions where odd behaviour patterns are liable to draw attention to the individual. Rather, the majority of cases were of depression and anxiety, conditions which are also under-detected in the general elderly population. Strikingly, only four of these twelve cases were known to psychiatric services.

Dementia in people with learning disabilities

Most people working in the learning disabilities field will have encountered dementia principally in the context of Down syndrome individuals. Such people are considerably more at risk of contracting Alzheimer-type dementia than their peers without Down syndrome. There is now considerable evidence that the brains of all people with Down syndrome aged 35 and over show the characteristic changes associated with Alzheimer-type dementia. Not all such individuals, however, show the behavioural and clinical symptoms described above. Research will no doubt eventually clarify why this should be so. In the mean time, it is important to emphasise that, despite the changes in the brain, *not* all people with Down syndrome *will* develop dementia.

Despite the high risk for Alzheimer's disease in Down syndrome, the absolute number of dementia sufferers without Down syndrome is probably greater. This is because a disproportionately large number of people with Down syndrome die before they reach age 50. In the Oldham study already referred to, for instance, only nine people over the age of 50 years with Down syndrome were found in a population of 105 individuals. Although the risk for the surviving people with Down syndrome is high, the non-Down population over 50 years of age is about ten times as large. These individuals have a dementia risk which is about the same as the general population. Unlike those with Down syndrome, these people are not likely to get dementia until they are in their 70s.

The prevalence rate from the total population study conducted in Oldham indicated 12 of the 105 to be suffering from dementia (11·4%). Of these twelve people, five were individuals with Down syndrome (of which there were only nine in the total population — an indication of the high risk for these individuals).

The combined prevalence for all diagnosable mental disorders in the Oldham study was 21% — a sizeable proportion of the total 50-plus population. In addition, their data on the physical health of this population (Moss *et al.*, 1993) showed that the group suffering from dementia had much poorer physical health than the group average. Health index measures indicated poorer scores for both chronic and acute physical disorders, particularly those involving the central nervous system and gastrointestinal functioning. Many of the individuals with a firm diagnosis of dementia showed deterioration in a wide variety of self-care and community skill domains.

This, coupled with their generally poor health, suggests that the needs of this particular group of people represents a major use of service resources.

With respect to the issues of dementia and learning disabilities, considerable attention has recently been given to the diagnosis of the condition in this population. A key publication has recently appeared on this subject and all persons involved in the process of diagnosis of dementia in people with learning disabilities should be aware of its contents. This publication — *Diagnosis of Dementia in Individuals with Intellectual Disability* (Aylward *et al.*, 1995) — proposes a set of standardised criteria for the diagnosis of dementia in people with learning disabilities for use by clinicians and researchers.

The issue of careful diagnosis is crucial because a number of conditions, many of them treatable, can mimic the early symptoms of dementia. These include depression, thyroid problems and sensory loss. A full clinical examination, and monitoring over at least six months, are necessary before a firm conclusion can be reached.

Some have questioned whether it is useful to be able to diagnose dementia, on the grounds that there is no cure anyway. There are two important replies to this. First, many conditions may be mistaken for dementia which, if properly diagnosed, may be reversed. Second, a cure for the condition, or at least the possibility of reducing risk of contracting the disorder, may eventually be discovered. With regard to diagnosis, there is an increasing awareness of the need to treat superimposed delirium and non-cognitive problems, such as depression, agitated behaviours, and psychotic symptoms, and to support the needs of caregivers with respite care programmes and community services. Substantial progress has also been made in understanding Alzheimer-type dementia and related disorders, and effective treatments based on new knowledge are on the horizon.

The first step is accurate diagnosis. Following this, the emphasis for people with learning disabilities is on care management across the various stages of the disease. The first authoritative statement on such management has recently been published in parallel to the paper on diagnosis noted above. *Practice Guidelines for the Clinical Assessment and Care Management of Alzheimer and other Dementias among Adults with Mental Retardation* (Janicki *et al.*, 1995) describes three steps in the overall strategy of dealing with dementia in a person with learning disabilities:

'*Step 1 – Understanding changes in normal ageing, being aware of risk factors, and recognising changes indicating onset of dementia.*

Step 2 – Conducting assessments and evaluation.

Step 3 – Instituting medical and care management.'

The guidelines go on to describe broad strategies for care management in the early, mid and late stage practices.

The pathway to care

The way by which people with learning disabilities come to the attention of psychiatric services is discussed in the section on **Detection and Assessment** (see **Chapter IV**). It is, however, of particular relevance in the context of ageing, because most of the psychiatric problems associated with ageing are the ones which are most likely to remain undetected — depression and anxiety disorders.

It is for this reason that only four of the twelve detected cases in the Oldham study had been recognised by psychiatric services. Not surprisingly, other studies have shown that older people with learning disabilities have a very low level of psychiatric service take-up. In one study, only ten referrals of older people with learning disabilities were made over a six-year period in a district of about 200,000 people (Ballinger, 1979). In eight of the ten instances the main reason for referral was behaviour disorder, sometimes associated with a failure in basic self-care. Ballinger also notes that the level of referral is low compared with non-disabled elderly people. A progressive fall in the proportion of people with psychiatric disorder as a function of age is also found elsewhere (Day, 1985).

Conclusion

In conclusion, it is clear that, while older people with learning disabilities may not demonstrate challenging behaviour to the same degree as younger populations, they nevertheless have mental health problems which need to be addressed. Staff training, both in relation to ageing and to the particular mental health problems of these older individuals is an essential part of service development in this respect. With regard to ageing, the reader's attention is drawn to the development of a comprehensive training pack which is shortly to be published by BILD, in conjunction with the White Top Research Centre at the University of Dundee, and the Hester Adrian Research Centre at the University of Manchester.

References and further reading

Aylward, E. H., Burt, D. B., Thorpe, L. U., Lai, F. & Dalton, A. J. (1995) *Diagnosis of Dementia in Individuals with Intellectual Disability*. Washington: American Association on Mental Retardation.

Ballinger, B. R. (1979) The elderly mentally handicapped in the community and a psychiatric service. *Apex: Journal of the British Institute of Mental Handicap, 7*, 40–41.

Day, K. A. (1985) Psychiatric disorder in the middle-aged and elderly mentally handicapped. *British Journal of Psychiatry, 147*, 660–667.

Day, K. A. & Jancar, J. (1994) Mental and physical health and ageing in mental handicap: a review. *Journal of Intellectual Disability Research, 38*, 241–256.

Gianturko, D. T. & Busse, E. W. (1978) Psychiatric problems encountered during a long-term study of normal ageing volunteers. In: A. D. Issacs (Ed.) *Studies in Geriatric Psychiatry*. Chichester: Wiley.

Hogg, J., Moss, S. & Cooke, D. (1988) *Ageing and Mental Handicap*. London: Chapman and Hall.

Holland, A. & Moss, S. C. (1996) Mental health problems related to ageing in people with learning disability. In: R. Jacoby (Ed.) *A Clinical Reader in Old-age Psychiatry*. Oxford: Oxford University Press.

Janicki, M. P., Heller, T., Seltzer, G. & Hogg, J. (1995) *Practice Guidelines for the Clinical Assessment and Care Management of Alzheimer and Other Dementias Among Adults with Mental Retardation*. Washington: American Association on Mental Retardation.

Moss, S. C. (1991) Age and functional abilities of people with a mental handicap: evidence from the Wessex mental handicap register. *Journal of Mental Deficiency Research, 35*, 430–445.

Moss, S. C., Goldberg, D., Patel, P. & Wilkin, D. (1993) Physical morbidity in older people with moderate, severe and profound mental handicap, and its relation to psychiatric morbidity. *Social Psychiatry and Psychiatric Epidemiology, 28*, 32–39.

Moss, S. C., Lambe, L., Hogg, J., & Lucchino, R. (1997) Managers' Reader 3: Physical and Mental Health. In: *Training Pack on Ageing and Learning Disability*. Kidderminster: BILD.

Patel, P., Goldberg, D. P., & Moss, S. C. (1993) Psychiatric morbidity in older people with moderate and severe learning disability (mental retardation). Part II: The prevalence study. *British Journal of Psychiatry, 163*, 481–491

Shamoian, C. A. (1985) Assessing depression in elderly patients. *Hospital and Community Psychiatry,* **36**, 338–339.

Shepherd, M., Cooper, B., Brown, A. C. (1966) *Psychiatric Illness in General Practice.* Oxford: Oxford University Press.

Sweeney, D. P. & Wilson, T. Y. (Eds.) (1979) *Double Jeopardy: The plight of ageing and aged developmentally disabled persons in mid-America.* Exceptional Child Center, Utah State University: Logan, Ut.

GLOSSARY

Compiled by Robert Winterhalder

ABC charts:	used by psychologists when assessing a problem behaviour. **A – Antecedents**, i.e. what leads up to the behaviour. **B – Behaviour**, i.e. the problem behaviour itself. **C – Consequences**, i.e. what follows the behaviour and how people react to it.
Absence seizures:	also known as *petit mal*; a sudden interference of consciousness occurs for a few seconds and motor activity (such as speech, eating or walking) is interrupted. The client may remain motionless and unresponsive during this time, but recovery is immediate and without confusion.
Acute:	of sudden onset and often short in duration.
Adaptive behaviour:	implies that an advantageous change has taken place regarding behaviour.
Aetiology:	the study of the causes of disease.
AIDS:	Acquired Immunodeficiency syndrome; this is a disorder that compromises the body's defence systems leading to repeated infections and malignancies (cancer). It is caused by a virus and transmitted by body fluids such as blood and semen.
Alzheimer's disease:	a progressive irreversible dementia of unknown origin (although research has shown a strong genetic component).

167

Amniocentesis:	transabdominal removal of fluid from the amniotic sac, which surrounds the fetus.
Anti-epileptic medication:	also called *anticonvulsants;* these are drugs used to treat epilepsy.
Anxiety disorder:	see under *neuroses.*
Assessments:	involve the appraisal of a situation or problem. When referring to psychiatry they take into account the physical, psychological and social components.
Atonic seizure:	a type of fit in which there is a sudden loss of tone and the client collapses; also known as a *'drop attack'.*
Autism:	a condition which usually manifests itself before the age of three, characterised by delay and deviation in the development of social relationships, verbal and non-verbal communication and imaginative activity, and a very restricted range of activities and interests.
Aura:	a peculiar sensation felt by the client immediately preceding an epileptic attack; for example, a sound, dizziness, or a churning sensation in the stomach.
Barbiturates:	a class of drugs used in the past as tranquillisers and sleeping pills, but no longer popular because of their high risk in overdose (they can be lethal) and their potential for addiction and abuse. Still sometimes used in very difficult cases of epilepsy.
Bart's test:	a screening test used in early pregnancy to detect those women at risk of having a pregnancy affected by Down syndrome.
Biological:	describes the science concerned with the phenomena of life and living organisms. Also used in the context of physical, non-psychological causes or treatments.

Breech:	commonly used in the term 'breech delivery', which means that the fetus is so positioned that the first part to present is the buttocks.
Brushfield spots:	whitish spots on the iris (the pigmented part of the eye) in people with Down syndrome.
Cataract:	a loss of transparency of the lens of the eye.
Cervical smear:	a thin specimen of cells obtained from the cervix (neck of the womb).
Challenging behaviour:	behaviour in an individual which is challenging to his or her carer. It is not necessarily due to a mental illness; for instance, challenging behaviour may result from frustration on the part of an individual with severe learning disabilities due to his or her inability to communicate their needs.
Chorionic villus sampling:	a technique to sample tissue from the placenta, which contains the same information as fetal tissue. This tissue is then analysed.
Chronic:	usually refers to disorders of long duration; for example, in chronic schizophrenia it means an episode that has been continuous for two years or more.
Clinical psychologist:	a professional concerned with the study of mental life and behaviour. Unlike psychiatrists, psychologists are not medically qualified (so, for example, they cannot prescribe medication).
Cognitive impairment:	a decline in the level of intellectual functioning — memory, concentration, communication, orientation, general intelligence and so on.
Complex partial seizure:	partial seizures in which consciousness is lost or impaired.

Counselling: the unburdening of problems, ventilation of feelings and discussion of current problems with a sympathetic and objective helper. Counselling is more 'practical', can involve giving advice, and does not go 'deeper', as in psychoanalysis where unconscious motives and dreams are explored.

Cri-du-chat: a chromosomal abnormality in which there is a deletion (i.e. a partial loss) in chromosome 5. This results in profound learning disabilities, failure to thrive and early death. The syndrome gains its name from the characteristic cat-like cry.

Cytomegalic inclusion virus: (CMV) a virus from the same family as the herpes virus. Infection of the mother when pregnant can lead to brain damage in the fetus and subsequent learning disabilities.

Defence mechanisms: one way of dealing with aspects of the self, which, if consciously experienced might give rise to unbearable anxiety, is by using a variety of defence mechanisms. Everybody needs and uses them — some defence mechanisms are healthy, others are not. Examples include denial and repression.

Delirium: a condition of extreme mental and usually motor excitement caused by a variety of physical illnesses. Delirium is marked by impaired consciousness, confusion and memory impairment, and is often accompanied by abnormal perceptions such as hallucinations.

Delusion: a false belief not amenable to persuasion or argument and out of keeping with the client's cultural and educational background.

Dementia: an acquired global impairment of intelligence, memory and personality without any impairment of consciousness. Most cases are progressive and irreversible.

Denial:	a defence mechanism (see defence mechanism) in which external reality is rejected and replaced by wish-fulfilling phantasy or behaviour.
Depersonalisation:	a change of self-awareness such that the person feels unreal. It is an unpleasant experience.
Depression:	a mental disorder characterised by a persistent lowering of mood and accompanied by various associated symptoms, such as alteration in sleep pattern, low self-esteem, diminished drive and so on.
Diabetes:	diseases that have in common the symptom of excessive production of urine. When used without qualification, the term refers to *diabetes mellitus* which is a metabolic disorder caused by a deficiency of insulin that leads to high sugar levels in the blood.
Didactic:	refers to instructing or teaching.
Down syndrome:	a syndrome caused by cells having an extra chromosome as a result of defects in early cell division. A chromosome contains genetic information.
Dysplasia:	abnormal development.
Emotional disorder:	disorders in which a mood, state (or feeling) such as fear or anxiety predominates.
Encephalitis:	inflammation of the brain.
Environmental causes:	causes that are external, i.e. in the environment.

Epicanthic fold: a fold of skin extending from the root of the nose to the near side of the eyebrow, thereby overlapping the medial angle of the eye. It is normal in fetal life but then usually disappears; it remains in Oriental peoples and in people with chromosomal disorders such as Down syndrome.

Epidemiology: the study of the prevalence and spread of disease in a community.

Epilepsy: an occasional, excessive and disorderly discharge in the brain which can lead to convulsions or reduction in consciousness. Sometimes it can also cause changes in behaviour, feelings and thoughts.

Experiential learning: learning by experience.

Explicit consent: consent that is plainly expressed and definite with no ambiguities; it is the opposite of implied consent.

Fragile-X syndrome: a cause of learning disabilities (mainly seen in males) due to a fragile site on the X chromosome. It can be inherited.

Guardianship: a section of *The Mental Health Act* which allows a person over the age of 16 to be placed under the supervision of a guardian. The application is made by the nearest relative or an approved social worker and is based on the recommendations of two doctors. Guardians have the power to require the person to reside at a specified place, attend specified places and times for treatment, education, training and so on, and allow access to doctors and approved social workers.

Generalised seizure: a form of epilepsy in which the epileptic disturbance and subsequent clinical signs involve both sides of the brain simultaneously from the onset of the attack. There are several types. Consciousness is impaired.

Generic psychiatrist:	a medical doctor who has been trained and has had experience in the diagnosis and treatment of psychiatric illness. The generic psychiatrist deals with mainstream adult psychiatry and does not specialise in one of its branches such as child psychiatry or forensic psychiatry.
Genetic causes:	causes which are a result of the influence of genes. A gene contains information which codes an individual's make-up and is passed on from generation to generation.
Hallucination:	this is a perception in the absence of a stimulus; for example, hearing a voice when there is no sound.
	Hearing a voice = perception
	No sound = absent stimulus.
	Hallucinations can occur in different forms; for example, visual, auditory, or to do with taste or smell.
HIV:	Human Immunodeficiency Virus — the cause of AIDS.
Hyperactivity:	general restlessness and excessive movement.
Hyperkinetic syndrome:	also known as attention deficit disorder; characterised by early onset, overactive behaviour, inability to persist with tasks, and marked inattention which is persistent and occurs in a number of situations.
Hypertension:	persistent high blood pressure.
Hypothyroid:	diminished production of thyroid hormones from the thyroid gland in the neck. This leads to an intolerance of cold, increased weight, constipation, slow pulse, a general slowing down in all physical and mental processes, and various psychiatric manifestations such as delirium, dementia, depression or psychosis.

Hypotonic:	reduced tension in a muscle; for example, a limb which has become 'floppy'.
Idiopathic:	denoting a disease of unknown cause.
Implicit consent:	consent is implied by lack of objection. Implicit consent is used all the time, especially in work with people with severe and profound learning disabilities. Examples include: changing soiled clothes, administering medication.
Incidence:	the number of new cases of a disease in a population over a period of time.
Intrauterine:	within the womb.
Irradiation atrophy:	wasting away of tissue following exposure to radiation.
Jacksonian seizure:	a type of partial seizure whose main characteristic is a jerking or spasm of muscles which 'marches' from a hand to an arm to a leg and the face.
Karyotyping:	a technique which allows the individual chromosomes in a nucleus to be separated and identified.
Learning disabilities:	developmental intellectual handicap, regardless of other handicaps, which means that a person requires extra help to experience an ordinary life, maintain good health, benefit from educational opportunities, maximise skills and minimise deficits. This term is currently used by the Department of Health in the UK. Other terms used with the same meaning are: learning difficulties (usually by Social Services Departments), developmental disability, mental handicap, mental retardation.

Lesch-Nyhan Syndrome:	an inherited disorder which results in the lack of an enzyme involved in the metabolism of purine. The subsequent accumulation of metabolites leads to learning disabilities, abnormal limb movements, self-mutilation and reduced life expectancy.
Leukaemia:	a progressive growth of certain blood cells (the white blood cells also known as leucocytes). It is malignant and often life-threatening although effective treatment is available for some subtypes. Leukaemia leads to severe vulnerability to infections, bleeding and anaemia.
Macro-orchidism:	enlarged testicles.
Makaton:	a form of sign language used with people who have learning disabilities.
Maladaptive:	often refers to types of behaviour that have been learned and which are inappropriate responses to the situation in question. Usually someone suffers as a result.
Meningitis:	inflammation of the membranes surrounding the brain or spinal cord.
Mental illness:	see **psychiatric disorders**.
Manic depression:	a disorder of mood which involves discrete episodes of depression and mania:
	Depression: the prevailing mood is one of sadness, varying from mild despondency to despair.
	Manic: the prevailing mood is one of elation, with high spirits, excitement and over-confidence. Some clients become very irritable.
	In both depression and mania, there are associated changes in thinking, behaviour, efficiency and physiological functioning. In very severe cases, the client may lose touch with reality, i.e. develop hallucinations or delusions.

Mental health:	the absence of a mental or behavioural disorder; mental health is a state of psychological well-being in which the individual has been able to integrate his or her more primitive drives with the norms expected by society.
Metabolism:	refers to the sum of the chemical changes occurring in tissues. It involves the creation of energy to: ● create building blocks for the body; ● eliminate waste products.
Monotherapy:	usually refers to drug treatment; monotherapy means that one drug only is being used to treat a disorder.
Multidisciplinary:	an approach in which all the agencies involved in a case take part in its management. Another term with the same meaning is *multiprofessional*.
Myoclonic seizure:	consists of brief jerks of a muscle group or several muscle groups which may be single or rapidly repetitive.
Neural tube defect:	this term is synonymous with **spina bifida**. In the early embryo, the nervous system is made up of a mass of nerve cells arranged as a tube — a defect in this neural tube leads to spina bifida.
Neuroses:	a group of psychiatric disorders in which contact with reality is maintained (i.e. there are no hallucinations or delusions). The symptoms are exaggerated forms of the normal reactions to stressful events; for example, in anxiety neurosis, a client presents with disabling levels of anxiety which are out of proportion to any trigger.

Obsessive compulsive: obsessions refer to words, ideas, images and the like, recognised by the client as his or her own, that intrude forcibly into the mind. Obsessions are unpleasant and often the client will try to resist them. Compulsions refer to repetitive, purposeful intentional behaviours performed in response to an obsession such as handwashing or checking.

Occiput: the back of the head.

Organic: physical or structural, i.e. not psychological or social.

Palpebral fissure: the space between the upper and lower eyelid.

Paranoid: a morbid and distorted view of the relationships between oneself and other people. Consequently, people who are paranoid are often suspicious.

Partial seizure: partial seizures are fits which initially involve only a small part of the brain. The characteristics of the fit reflect the part of the brain involved.

Perinatal: this terms refers to the periods before, during and after the time of birth, i.e. from the 28th week of pregnancy to the seventh day after delivery.

Phenylketonuria: an inherited disorder which results in a lack of an enzyme (a substance which helps metabolise other substances) involved in the metabolism of an amino acid (phenylalanine). The subsequent accumulation of phenylalanine leads to brain damage, learning disabilities, epilepsy and eczema. It can be treated by excluding phenylalanine from the diet.

Phobia:	an irrational abnormal fear in relation to a thing, situation or stimulus which normally would not evoke such fear. The client realises that the fear is irrational; however, the phobia often leads to avoidance of the feared stimulus or situation.
Pica:	the persistent eating of non-nutritional substances including paper, dirt, hair, paint and cigarette stubs.
Postnatal:	refers to the period after childbirth.
Prader-Willi syndrome:	a genetic condition which includes insatiable appetite, gross overeating, obesity, under-developed genitalia, pica, skin-picking, irritability and stubbornness.
Prefertilisation:	refers to events which occur prior to the joining of the male sperm to the female egg.
Prevalence:	the number of existing cases of a disease in a given population at a specific time.
Prospective consent:	this occurs when, for example, relatives sign forms allowing their son or daughter to go riding, boating on the river, or to have an operation. Prospective consent has no standing in law.
Psychological:	refers to the mind and its various processes. There are various components, including thoughts, feelings and memories, and the observed behaviour that results.
Psychomotor:	refers to a combination of mental and behavioural events. For example: **psychomotor retardation**; this is often seen in depression where both mental processes and body movements are slowed down **psychomotor epilepsy**; this is an old term which describes a type of epilepsy with both behavioural and mental features.

Psychopathic disorder:	a type of personality disorder in which there is a deeply ingrained, maladaptive pattern of behaviour, recognisable by adolescence and continuing throughout most of adult life. The individual or society suffers. Psychopathic disorder is not a result of learning disabilities, psychosis, neurosis or any other form of psychiatric illness. The characteristics of this disorder are: self-centredness with little or no regard for the rights of others — immediate satisfaction of desire is imperative, the individual acting violently if frustrated — and associated with lack of conscience or guilt; and inability to learn from previous experience.
Psychotherapist:	a person, usually a psychiatrist or clinical psychologist, professionally trained in psycho-therapy which is a form of treatment used in mental disorders. Psychotherapy attempts to understand current problems in terms of past experiences.
Psychiatric disorder:	a significant behavioural or psychological pattern occurring in a person that is associated with distress, disability (an impairment in one or more areas of functioning) or with a significant risk of suffering death, pain, disability or important loss of freedom. It does not encompass an expected response to a particular event — such as the loss of a loved one — nor does it include religious, sexual or political deviant behaviours.
Psychological presentation:	usually refers to looking at a problem in psychological terms.
Psychoses:	a group of mental disorders characterised by an inability to recognise reality and to distinguish it from subjective experience. It is often accompanied by lack of insight (an awareness of one's own mental condition). As a result hallucinations, delusions and so on may occur.

Public sanctions:	this term can be used in various ways but when used in an ethical sense it means 'anything approved by society and which makes a rule of conduct binding'.
Pyrexia:	fever.
Reminiscence:	the act of recalling a past event, i.e. a memory.
Risk taking:	risk is defined as the chance or likelihood of harm, injury or loss. Risk taking is a term often used in the context of assessing the advantages and disadvantages of a course of action with regards to risk.
Rubella:	German measles — an infection caused by a virus which, if contracted by a woman in the first three months of pregnancy, can lead to brain damage, learning disabilities, cataracts, deafness and heart defects in the newborn.
Schizophrenia:	a group of psychiatric disorders characterised by disordered thinking processes, hallucinations, delusions (false beliefs not amenable to persuasion or argument and out of keeping with the client's cultural and educational background), bizarre behaviour and social withdrawal. Not all of these characteristics have to be present to make the diagnosis.
Sacral agenesis:	Present at birth, sacral agenesis consists of absence of formation of the sacral bone. It is associated with malformations of the intestine and bladder and requires major surgery.
Simian crease:	a single groove across the palm of the hand seen in people with Down syndrome.

Simple partial seizures:	these fits initially involve only a small part (focus) of the brain. If there is no alteration of consciousness they are termed '*simple*'; if consciousness is impaired or lost, they are termed '*complex*'.
Social:	pertaining to society; often refers to the influence of society.
Spina bifida:	a defect in the spinal column, consisting of the absence of the vertebral arches, through which the membranes surrounding the spinal cord, with or without spinal cord tissue, may protrude.
Status epilepticus:	a condition in which one major attack of epilepsy succeeds another with little or no intermission.
Stereotypies:	repetitive primitive and self-stimulatory movements such as body-rocking and head-shaking.
Stigma:	to be devalued by society because of one's beliefs, origins and the like, or, in the context of medicine, because of an associated physical or mental disorder: for example, the stigma of epilepsy or schizophrenia.
Stress:	refers to factors (called stressors) which tax individuals' coping mechanisms to their limits and which, if long or severe enough, can lead to disorganised behaviour, dysfunction or disease. Examples include: **physical stressors**, such as infection **psychological stressors**, such as bereavement **social stressors**, such as homelessness.
Stroke:	the sudden onset of neurological signs and symptoms due to problems with the blood supply to the brain.

181

Spurious consent: this implies a 'double negative'; for example: 'We will not act unless we hear from you to the contrary...' In such situations, consent is implied from a non-response.

Syphilis: an infection caused by a bacterium and transmitted by direct contact – usually through sexual intercourse. Infection in a pregnant woman can lead to miscarriage or fetal brain damage.

Therapeutic intervention: any form of treatment — such as medication, surgery, counselling, or moving to improved accommodation — which has as its aim the cure of an illness or at least a reduction in suffering.

Tonic-clonic seizures: also known as *grand mal*; an attack may start with a cry and the client will fall and stiffen (the tonic phase) after which the clonic phase occurs — this involves convulsive movements usually of all four limbs. This phase may last several minutes and is succeeded by a phase of unconsciousness, confusion or sleep.

Toxin: a noxious or poisonous substance.

Toxoplasmosis: an infection often transmitted by cats which, in a pregnant woman, can lead to miscarriage or brain damage in the fetus.

Trisomy 21: the human cell normally has 46 chromosomes: 22 pairs numbered 1 to 22, plus two sex chromosomes — two Xs in a female, one X and one Y in a male. Trisomy 21 means that there are 47 chromosomes: instead of a pair of chromosome 21 there are 3 chromosomes 21. This is one of the causes of Down syndrome.

Tuberous sclerosis: an inherited disorder which may lead to learning disabilities. It is characterised by epilepsy and skin lesions.

　　　182

Turner's syndrome:	a sex-chromosome abnormality in girls where one X chromosome is absent. The child is likely to be short, stocky, have a webbed neck and be infertile with absent menstrual periods.
Ultrasound:	an investigation which uses high-frequency sound waves to form images of internal body structures.
Valid consent:	this exists when a competent client is given information which he or she understands and when he or she is then able to make a positive decision voluntarily. If any of the above criteria are missing, valid consent does not exist.
Vulnerability:	a susceptibility to suffering, loss, disease and so on.

CONTRIBUTORS

Sarah Bernard
Consultant Psychiatrist in
Child Learning Disability
The Maudsley Hospital
Denmark Hill
London SE5 BAZ

Nick Bouras
Professor of Psychiatry
in Learning Disabilites
Guy's, King's and St Thomas'
School of Medicine
and
Institute of Psychiatry
King's College London
and
Consultant Psychiatrist
South London and Maudsley NHS Trust
Estia Centre
Munro
Guy's Hospital
London SE1 3RR

Jill Bradshaw
Speech and Language Therapist
Teaching Fellow
The Tizard Centre
University of Canterbury
Canterbury
Kent CT2 7LZ

Ella Brent
Clinical Psychologist in Training
University College London
Phillips House
Gower Street
London WC1E 6BT

David Brook
Consultant Psychiatrist
South London and Maudsley NHS Trust
and
Honorary Senior Lecturer
Guy's, King's and St Thomas'
School of Medicine
King's College
Estia Centre
Munro
Guy's Hospital
London SE1 3RR

Helen Costello
Research Fellow
South London and Maudsley NHS Trust
Estia Centre
Munro
Guy's Hospital
London SE1 3RR

Anna Eliatamby
Psychologist
Department of Psychology
St Brendan's Hospital
PO Box DV501
Devonshire
Bermuda DVBX

Geraldine Holt
Consultant Psychiatrist
South London and Maudsley NHS Trust
and
Senior Lecturer
Guy's, King's and St Thomas'
School of Medicine
King's College
Estia Centre
Munro
Guy's Hospital
London SE1 3RR

Andrea Hughes
Principal Psychologist
Oxleas NHS Trust
Lodge Hill
London SE2

John Gavilan
Consultant Psychiatrist in Learning
Disabilities
Hounslow and Spelthorne NHS Trust
1a Walpole Road
Staines
Middlesex
TW18 1ED

Shaun Gravestock
Consultant Psychiatrist
Oxleas NHS Trust
and
Honorary Senior Lecturer
Guy's, King's and St Thomas'
School of Medicine
King's College
Estia Centre
Munro
Guy's Hospital
London SE1 3RR

Theresa Joyce
Consultant Psychologist
South London and Maudsley NHS Trust
and
Honorary Senior Lecturer
Guy's, King's and St Thomas'
School of Medicine
King's College
19–21 Brownhill Road
London SE6 2HG

Yan Kon
Consultant Psychiatrist in
Learning Disabilities
South Tees Community and Mental
Health NHS Trust
Oakwood
22 Belview Grove
Middlesborough TS4 2PX

Susan Macdonald
Teaching Fellow in Applied Psychology
The Tizard Centre
University of Kent at Canterbury
Canterbury
Kent CT2 7LZ

Steve Moss
Senior Lecturer
Section of Psychiatric Nursing
Institute of Psychiatry
Health Service Research Centre
King's College
London SE5 8AZ

Barley Oliver
Consultant Psychologist
South London and Maudsley NHS Trust
19–21 Brownhill Road
London SE6 2HG

Helen Prosser
Hester Adrian Research Centre
University of Manchester
Oxford Road
Manchester M13 9PL

Jeremy Turk
Senior Lecturer in Child and Adolescent
Psychiatry
St George's Hospital Medical School
Crammer Terrace
London SW17 0RE

Robert Winterhalder
Consultant Psychiatrist
Guy's Hospital
and
Honorary Senior Lecturer
Guy's, King's and St Thomas'
School of Medicine
King's College
Estia Centre
Munro
Guy's Hospital
London SE1 3RR

INDEX

index

drugs, therapeutic 41–3, 53–67, 101–2
DSM *see* Diagnostic and Statistical Manual of
    Mental Disorders
duty of care 121

echoed speech 149–50
education 50, 132, 134, 137, 138–40
electroconvulsive therapy (ECT) 42
Eliatamby, A. 45–51
Emerson, E. 70, 105
emotion
    dementia 160
    psychotherapy 37–8, 39, 40
    trauma 75
emotional disorders 17–25, 27–36, 58, 136–7
    see also autism; challenging behaviour;
    neuroses
emotional intelligence 7–8
employment 101
environment 73, 76, 77–8, 89
Epanutin *see* phenytoin
epilepsy 97–103, 138
    anti-epileptics 59, 61–6, 101–2
    antipsychotics 56
    challenging behaviour 72
    differential mortality 158
Epilim *see* sodium valproate
ethical issues 125–8
ethosuximide (Zarontin) 63
explicit consent 120
expression 148–9

facial expression 148, 149
families
    adjustment 9–12
    aetiology of dual diagnosis 135, 137
    children's needs 131, 134
    emotional disorders 18
fertilisation *see* prefertilisation
finance 127
Firth, H. 107
Fleming, I. 106
Fragile-X syndrome 23, 92–5
functional analysis 46–7, 48, 50, 76

gabapentin (Neurontin) 64
Gavilan, J. 111–29
general practitioners (GPs) 27–8
generic names, medication 54
genetic factors, learning disabilities 89, 92–5
gestures 147, 148
Gould, J. 150
GPs *see* general practitioners

Gravestock, S. 7–15, 17–26
grief *see* bereavement
group psychotherapy 39
guardianship 114–15, 116

hallucinations 54
Hatton, C. 105
Hester Adrian Research Centre 34–5
Holt, G. 1, 83–8, 105–9
home-based intervention 86
Hughes, A. 111–29
hyperactivity 23
hyperkinetic disorder 139–40
hypnotics 60–1, 63
hypomania 54, 58

ICD *see* International Classification of Diseases
illness *see* physical illness
imagination 151–2
implicit consent 120
individuals
    adjustment 7–9
    aetiology of dual diagnosis 135
    stress reduction 107–8
insight 8
insomnia 61
institutionalisation 5–6
    see also deinstitutionalisation
instruments, psychiatric assessment 34–6, 47,
    76
intelligence 3, 7–8
Intelligence Quotient (IQ) 3
'interest sharing' 147
interests, restricted 151–2
International Classification of Diseases (ICD)
    31–2
interpersonal relationships 100, 125–6
intervention *see* therapeutic intervention
interviews, diagnostic 33
intrauterine aetiology, learning disabilities **90**,
    91, 95
IQ *see* Intelligence Quotient

Jancar, J. 161
Joyce, T. 69–81

Knapp, M. 107
Kon, Y. 53–67
Kroese, B. S. 106

La Vigna, G. W. 48
labelling, learning disabilities 3
lamotrogine (Lamictal) 64

